Praise for LIVING AT THE END OF LIFE

"As a hospice nurse for 16 years, [Karen Whitley] Bell understands the concept of a 'good death.' A daily witness to fatal illness and end-of-life moments, Bell's powerful message is aimed at making sure the final months or days of a patient are well lived, marked by peace, comfort, and a chance to say good-bye. Illustrating the tenets and benefits of palliative care with firsthand accounts of her patients, Bell manages, as stated by American Academy of Hospice and Palliative Medicine co-founder Charles G. Sasser in his foreword, to place readers 'at bedsides during one of the most intimate of life's dramas.' As such, she delivers a wealth of useful information on pain management, choosing a hospice and general day-to-day care giving in a powerful, hard-to-forget way. Straightforward and empathetic, with an easy-to-navigate style, Bell details what to expect in both physical and spiritual terms, including practical considerations as well as ways to find closure and cope with loss."

—*Publishers Weekly* (Starred Review)

"This book is rich in stories, generous, full of wisdom, organized to serve the needs of those facing their own final journeys or those of their loved ones."

—Patrick Clary, MD, author of *Dying for Beginners*

"This book enables you to pick and choose what you're able to face, allowing you time to process, revisit, and come to terms at all levels: physical, spiritual, and mental. Even if you're not facing the end of life process with a loved one, this book will assist you in considering all that is valuable in the moment."

—Melissa Joseph, author of *Moments with Baxter*

"Nuggets of wisdom and satisfying aha's support and inspire the reader. Providing explicit practical guidance, this treasure trove is the perfect offering for anyone interested in accessing hopes and strengths and confronting and diminishing personal fears both prior to and after a death. This book should be in the waiting rooms of every hospital and clinician's office, and shelved in a prominent and accessible place in everyone's personal library. If there were a 'textbook' for compassionate care—for authenticity in relationship—this blend of the personal, practical and poetic would be it."

—Sandra Bertman, PhD, author of
Facing Death: Images, Insights and Interventions

"Many people are afraid of dying and don't know what to expect in the final months and days of life. This important book takes aim at ameliorating those fears by shedding light on some of the most common concerns and revealing what should be expected from the healthcare system."

—Scott A. Irwin, MD, PhD, Director, Palliative Care
Psychiatry Program, The Institute for Palliative
Medicine at San Diego Hospice

"*Living at the End of Life* is a wonderful read that says what so many long to hear when first hearing the words that upset their worlds . . . Bravo! Those who read it will feel empowered to Live right up until they die!"

—Sherry E. Showalter, PhD, author of
Healing Heartaches, Stories of Loss and Life

"This book sees the person and guides them gracefully to the opportunity to heal . . . I was continually touched by the tenderness and the preciousness of the stories shared."

—Loren Spagnuolo, Drishti Point Radio

"Hospice nurse Karen Whitley Bell has seen every type of emotion in her 16 years of assisting both the dying and their families. In the book *Living at the End of Life*, Bell answers the most common questions, including how to get started with hospice care, what to expect, ensuring your final plans are carried out, and dozens of other hard-to-express questions that need answering."

—*Quincy Herald-Whig*

Living
at the End *of* Life

A Hospice Nurse Addresses the Most Common Questions

Karen Whitley Bell, RN

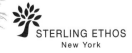

STERLING ETHOS
New York

For All the Families, and For B—

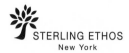

STERLING ETHOS
New York

An Imprint of Sterling Publishing
387 Park Avenue South
New York, NY 10016

STERLING ETHOS and the distinctive Sterling logo are registered trademarks of
Sterling Publishing Co., Inc.

ISBN 978-1-4027-6838-5 (hardcover)
ISBN 978-1-4027-8728-7 (paperback)
ISBN 978-1-4027-7673-1 (ebook)

Library of Congress Cataloging-in-Publication Data
Bell, Karen Whitley.
Living at the end of life: a hospice nurse addresses the most common questions/Karen Whitley Bell.
p. cm.
Includes bibliographical references and index.
ISBN 978-1-4027-6838-5
1. Hospice care. 2. Hospice nurses. I. Title.
RT87.T45B45 2009
362.17'56--dc22

2009023570

Distributed in Canada by Sterling Publishing
c/o Canadian Manda Group, 165 Dufferin Street
Toronto, Ontario, Canada M6K 3H6
Distributed in the United Kingdom by GMC Distribution Services
Castle Place, 166 High Street, Lewes, East Sussex, England BN7 1XU
Distributed in Australia by Capricorn Link (Australia) Pty. Ltd.
P.O. Box 704, Windsor, NSW 2756, Australia

For information about custom editions, special sales, and premium and corporate purchases, please
contact Sterling Special Sales at 800-805-5489 or specialsales@sterlingpublishing.com.

Manufactured in the United States of America

2 4 6 8 10 9 7 5 3

www.sterlingpublishing.com

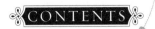

CONTENTS

Chapters can be read in any order, based on your needs. You do not need to read the entire guide. Read only what you feel will be of value to you.

❄ FOREWORD ❄

FOR MOST OF US, FACING INCURABLE, life-threatening illness in ourselves or a loved one is a terrifying experience. Although we may have considered the possibility, it is not something we can actively plan for, and its effects usually take us by surprise. There are a number of "how to" books on the market filled with practical hints to guide newcomers encountering life's final chapter. In the category of end-of-life literature are autobiographies of people stricken with illness, philosophical and spiritual musings, and scientific textbooks. As the population ages and chronic illness becomes more commonplace, self-help survival guides are added to the collection.

Living at the End of Life is much more than a self-help manual. By inserting real-life dialogue into the extensive list of issues to be faced, Karen Whitley Bell places the reader at bedsides during one of the most intimate of life's dramas. Reading about what others have experienced and the common questions they have asked gives a firsthand feel to the narrative. People grappling with illness and their caregivers often find themselves overwhelmed with questions about a future they are afraid to contemplate, and don't know how or what to ask. This book asks those questions, and the follow-up answers—provided in the context of discussions among givers and receivers of care—offer reassurance, encouragement, and hope.

The language people use with each other and with their health care professionals about dying often lead to the most intimate and profound of conversations. After nearly thirty years in hospice and palliative care, I continue to be awed by how people facing life-threatening illness describe their plight, as well as both the healing and damaging potential of the language health care professionals choose in end-of-life conversations. A key to excellence in palliative care is the recognition that when it comes to the art of dying, they are the teachers and we the students. Palliative specialists provide expertise in comfort and pain and symptom management, and they receive in return remarkable insights into the illness experience, provided by the only ones who really know what it's like. We are all wounded in some way and, in the care of those with incurable, terminal illness, the distinction between givers and receivers of care becomes blurred.

Ego chill is a phrase used to describe the shock of realization that our nonexistence is possible. Accompanying the shock is an almost universal desire to cling to life at any cost and to desperately seek, if not a cure, at least a delay to the end of existence. *Curative hope* describes this all-consuming urge to fight, to resist, to be rescued from, and not to think about, the unthinkable. Although modern medicine is grand, the energy and time invested in curative hope often lead both seekers and providers of health care down paths they, in retrospect, wish they had never chosen.

Making the transition from curative to *palliative hope* is one of the hardest challenges of life's final chapter. With palliative hope, the frame of reference shifts from hope for a physical cure to hope for *healing,* a word that encompasses much more than what happens to the body. In palliative hope, healing—which can take place in the midst of continual physical decline, even unto death—has to do with a restoration of wholeness to mind and spirit and to relationships, as well as a restoration of coherence to one's life story. Here we were, telling one story with our lives, and along comes this unanticipated and uninvited illness that wrecks the story we were creating for ourselves. Now, in a time frame beyond our control, we have to create a new story, with the illness in it, and decide—here we still have some control—if we will ultimately be defined by the illness or by some greater meaning of our choosing.

Palliative hope is all about that choice. It's about bringing closure, completing tasks, recognizing that our loved ones can make it without us, and celebrating the gifts we have given and the example we have provided that will help them accomplish this. It's all about love, forgiveness, saying good-bye, and making sure that any regrets are dealt with. Unfortunately, time constraints in life's final chapter don't always provide opportunities for both curative and palliative endeavors. We usually have to choose.

This book considers what it might be like to choose palliative hope.

The stories of the various aspects of this experience found here reveal the different ways people and families face their illness, with examples of how these conversations may go and the remarkable healing impact of words carefully chosen. When agendas differ, conflict is common. But when discussion time is allowed for personal values and goals of care to be clarified, as demonstrated in these narratives, tensions quickly dissolve and everyone finds common ground.

People who are dying want, more than anything, to have caregivers who are both loving and competent. Their caregivers want, more than anything, to provide loving, competent care. And their health care professionals seek the skills and insights necessary to provide both state-of-the-art pain and symptom management and to serve as compassionate witnesses to the incredible final chapter they are invited to share. This book has much to offer all three.

—Dr. Charles G. Sasser, MD, FAAHPM, FACP

❋ INTRODUCTION ❋

What's going to happen? How will we manage? There are things I still want to do. I'm afraid . . .

So begins this journey. It is a time of challenge, of concerns, but also an opportunity to explore and rediscover the fuller, richer meaning of life.

This book offers guidance to individuals and their loved ones by sharing the experiences of others who have traveled this extraordinary road. Their stories offer different perspectives, impart knowledge, and reveal possibilities. Their lessons offer the opportunity to discover our own path to cope with decline, realize meaning, attain closure, rediscover hope, and achieve peace.

It also includes suggestions, discussion questions, lists, and other resources to help you and your loved ones develop your own solutions to reflect your unique needs and values.

What does it mean to undertake this journey? You alone can discover that answer. You alone will choose your path.

What This Guide Offers

- ❋ Insights into meaning and hope, offered by those who have made this journey
- ❋ An understanding of the opportunities and challenges of this time in life
- ❋ Practical caregiving instructions
- ❋ Insights into emotional and spiritual issues
- ❋ Ideas for creating meaningful conversations
- ❋ Guidance to address conflict and unresolved issues
- ❋ An explanation of common physical changes
- ❋ Suggestions to maximize energy and mobility
- ❋ Ideas for adapting to a changing appetite
- ❋ Information on common pain medications, and guidance for medication management

- An explanation of hospice and the services it offers
- Safety tips
- An exploration of care settings outside the home
- Descriptions of supportive therapies to improve comfort and quality of life
- Suggestions for managing care if hospice service is not available
- Lists of resources for additional information or support

How to Use This Guide

Some chapters address the needs of individuals coping with declining health. Other chapters focus on the challenges faced by loved ones and caregivers. Many chapters offer information that may be helpful to everyone involved in the end of life transition. You do not need to read the entire guide. Read only what you feel will be of value to you.

To locate the information you need, read "How This Guide Is Organized" below, then turn to the Table of Contents and select the topic of interest to you. Chapters can be read in any order.

Next, read the brief chapter, which explores the practical concerns and emotional factors unique to that issue. In most cases, both must be addressed to achieve a real solution. Then review the list of suggestions, tools, or discussion questions at the end of that chapter to help you develop your own solution.

Explanation of Terms

For each of us, the word *family* holds a different meaning. In this guide, *family* applies to whomever you, the reader, define as your family, and may include close friends, a partner, relatives, pets, or other loved ones.

Just as we define our family, we also define our own *spirituality*. In this guide, *spirituality* refers to how we view ourselves, our sense of being within a broader context. Regardless of our culture, beliefs, or religious traditions, we ask common questions and encounter common phenomena that may influence our views of our existence. This guide presents an objective account, allowing you to gain insights into these experiences while applying your own beliefs to determine meaning for you.

In keeping with hospice practices, this guide does not advocate any specific religious points of view.

Consciousness can mean both "active consciousness," what we commonly think of as being awake, and "awareness," which can occur without our being awake.

How This Guide Is Organized

Part I: What Will Happen? The Spiritual Journey

This section offers information that may be helpful to individuals coping with declining health, their loved ones, and caregivers.

In this section you'll learn about the special awareness, communications, and visions some people experience before passing. Information about these occurrences is offered to help you understand what you may experience, or what your loved ones might witness during your final days. These occurrences happen frequently and are well documented in professional hospice literature. They are consistent in theme, regardless of the cultural, spiritual, or religious practices of those who experience them. They may be the result of the subconscious emerging; they may have a spiritual origin, or they may have other causes. No one knows why they occur, or what they mean. Only you can decide what they might mean for you.

Part II: What Will Happen? The Physical Journey

This section offers information that may be helpful to individuals coping with declining health.

In this section you'll learn what this journey may be like for you. You'll learn what physical and emotional changes you may experience, and discover tools to cope with these changes. You'll also learn about some of the legal and practical issues you and your loved ones may face, and ways to address them. Most chapters are followed by a list of suggestions, tools, or other resources to help you develop a solution that reflects your unique needs and values.

Part III: Caregiving as a Family: How Do We Manage?

This section offers information that may be helpful for loved ones and caregivers. Individuals coping with declining health may find value in some of this material, as well.

In this section you'll learn how to adapt to physical decline. You'll find suggestions to maximize mobility, energy, and safety; advice for adapting to a changing appetite; tips for gathering and organizing help; and information about available resources, including hospice. You'll learn about how to manage communication and minimize conflict within your family. You'll also find guidance for selecting a care facility, if caregiving at home is no longer possible. Each chapter is followed by extensive checklists and other tools for quick and easy reference.

Part IV: Closure: Will I Die a "Good" Death?

This section offers information that may be of value to individuals seeking meaning as their life nears its end, and to family members supporting a loved one through this process. Not all chapters will be relevant to your situation, so read only what you feel applies to you.

In this section you'll explore some of the challenges people may face as they review their life and search for meaning. You'll discover how others have addressed these issues, and how they resolved them. You'll find practical tips as well as discussion questions to help you explore your own feelings to achieve resolution, meaning, and peace.

Part V: For Loved Ones and Caregivers: Sharing the Final Days

This section offers information that may be especially helpful for loved ones and caregivers. To better understand and prepare for the issues presented in this section, consider reading these chapters before the final days.

In this section you'll learn how to care for someone in the final days. You'll find information about physical changes that may occur, and what these changes mean. You'll learn how to keep your loved one comfortable, and how to recognize if she's comfortable, even if she can't tell you how she feels. You'll also discover what you can do at the time of passing to honor your loved one and create a special memory, if you choose.

Part VI: How Will I Go On? Coping with Loss

This section offers information that may be helpful to loved ones beginning their grieving process.

This section provides an introduction to the journey of grief, an ever-changing process that each of us experiences in our own way. You'll learn about common physical and emotional changes you may experience, as well as tools and resources to help you understand and cope.

Part VII: Living

This section offers information that may be helpful to anyone affected by loss, and can be read at any time during this journey.

This section relates some of the remarkable lessons I've been offered about life and living from individuals and families who have shared their journey with me. I share their courage, grace, and wisdom with you, in hopes that you, too, will discover your own path to meaning, hope, and peace.

I am grateful to the many families I've been privileged to serve and learn from in my fifteen years as a hospice nurse, providing care and support in homes, hospice residences, and hospitals. The events shared in this guide are actual experiences. One chapter, "What If We Don't Have Hospice Care?" is a composite of two families' similar experiences. To respect their privacy, names and other identifying details have been changed.

Nothing worth doing is complete in our lifetime,
Therefore, we are saved by hope.
Nothing true or beautiful or good makes complete sense in any immediate
context of history,
Therefore, we are saved by faith.
Nothing we do, however virtuous, can be achieved alone,
Therefore, we are saved by love.
No virtuous act is ever as virtuous from the standpoint of our friend or
foe as from our own,
Therefore we are saved by the final form of love which is forgiveness.

—*Reinhold Niebuhr*

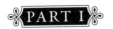

PART I

What Will Happen?
The Spiritual Journey

This section offers information that may be helpful to individuals coping with declining health, their loved ones, and caregivers.

In this section you'll learn about the special awareness, communications, and visions some people experience before passing. Information about these occurrences is offered to help you understand what you may experience, or what your loved ones might witness during your final days. These occurrences happen frequently and are well documented in professional hospice literature. They are consistent in theme, regardless of the cultural, spiritual, or religious practices of those who experience them. They may be the result of the subconscious emerging; they may have a spiritual origin, or they may have other causes. No one knows why they occur, or what they mean. Only you can decide what they might mean for you.

What Will It Be Like?
An Overview of the End-of-Life Journey

Will I Be Alone?
Will Others Be with You in Your Final Days or Hours?

Will I Choose My Time?
Does the Mind or Spirit Influence When We Pass?

Will I Be Aware?
The Possibility of Consciousness, Even If We're Not Awake or Responsive

I Had This Dream . . .
A Description of Common Dream Themes

❈ WHAT WILL IT BE LIKE? ❈
An Overview of the End-of-Life Journey

Eddie

"WHAT WILL IT BE LIKE?" EDDIE ASKS, holding my hand.

I gaze at him, looking for signs of fear, but see none. Instead, I see a quiet acceptance, wisdom, and a grace rarely found in this time and culture in which we live. Most of us live our lives in haste, in pursuit of goals, in denial: "I must hurry. I must have more. It will not happen to me."

And yet it does happen, to all of us. In that realization there are both questions and choices. In the months, weeks, days, hours, and moments that remain, what will this journey be like? *What will I say to those I love? How will they remember me? Will I suffer? Will I find closure? Will I be at peace?*

Eddie looks at me, his hand holding mine, waiting, asking, what will it be like?

I think about the young man I've only just met. Labeled as "developmentally delayed" at an early age, his mother abandoned him and he became a ward of the state, growing up in group homes, making his own family, forming deep friendships bonded by his disarming smile, infectious laugh, and generous spirit. He ambled through life at his own pace, taking time to discover what most would overlook. He found joy in giving, happiness in making others smile.

Over the years I've come to realize that we die in much the same way as we live. If we have been open, generous, and kind in our living, we will make this final passage with that same sense of peacefulness. If we've spent our lives struggling for control, always fearful, always holding tight to what we have, then in death we will also struggle—against the loss of control, against the unknown, against letting go. But even then, in our final months, weeks, and days, we have a choice.

"I believe you will be peaceful," I say. "The people here at the foster home will take good care of you, and nurses like me will come see you to ask how you're feeling. We'll all work together to make sure you stay comfortable."

Eddie blinks but makes no other response, and I continue. "You'll begin to sleep more. You won't have all the energy you used to have. At some point, you may want to just stay in bed, and that's okay. They'll help you. They'll bring things to you."

I watch his face, looking for change, for fear, but see none. "You won't feel like eating as much as you used to. That's your body telling you it hasn't got the energy to digest it. At some point you'll probably want to eat just a little bit at a time. And when you do feel like eating, it will probably be things like pudding or custards or ice cream. That's okay. The people here will understand why you don't feel like eating. They'll know that it's not because you don't like the food, or don't appreciate that they brought it. They'll know you're not eating much because your body just isn't up to it anymore.

"You'll probably want to spend more time alone, just being quiet, not watching television or reading, or being with visitors. You may just want to lie in bed, or recline in a chair, resting with your eyes closed.

"In those quiet times you may think about all the people you care about, all the good memories you share with them, how they make you happy, and how good you feel that they're a part of your life. And when you think about them, know that you've made them happy, too."

A tear escapes from the corner of his eye. He does not wipe it away.

"You might also think about sad things, like how much you'll miss your friends, and about all the things you've dreamed of doing, but now won't be able to. It's okay to be sad." I squeeze his hand. "It's okay to cry. Sometimes just letting all that emotion out, just letting go instead of trying to hold it all in can make you feel a lot better."

I wait, wondering. Is this enough? Or does he want to know more? I feel a slight squeezing of his hand around mine. I nod and continue.

"As time goes by, you'll sleep most of the time. Sometimes you might dream about your old friends, people you haven't seen in a long time. Then you might begin to dream about going on a trip. And finally, you may dream about the people you love who have already passed away. They'll be good dreams. You won't be afraid.

"When the time is very close, you might feel a surge of energy. Some people do. More likely, you'll be deeply asleep, but I think you'll be aware of what's happening around you, even if you can't respond.

"And I think, Eddie, when you're ready, you'll peacefully let go and make your journey to whatever is next."

Another tear spills from the corner of his eye. "What *is* next?" he asks.

"What do *you* think is next?"

He shrugs. "I don't know. . . ."

I smile. "I don't, either. But I think whatever is waiting for you, Eddie, whatever is next, I think it will be wonderful. I think it will be beautiful. I think it will be peaceful."

He closes his eyes. For a long time we sit quietly together, his hand holding mine. Then he opens his eyes. His gaze travels to some distant place, far beyond me. "Will I get to say good-bye to everybody?"

"Yes, when you're ready."

Slowly, he nods. His gaze returns to that distant place. His mouth forms a small smile.

What is important is not what happens to us, but how we respond to what happens to us.

—Jean-Paul Sartre

THE JOURNEY

For each person, this journey is unique. You may experience some or all of these changes. Additional information can be found throughout this guide.

Months Before Passing

- Withdrawal and reflection
- Decreased appetite, changes in food preferences
- Decreased energy
- Increased need for sleep
- Vivid dreams
- Need for some assistance with personal care

Weeks Before Passing

- Minimal appetite; prefer easily digested foods
- Further increase in the need for sleep
- Increased weakness
- Increased need for assistance with care

Days Before Passing

- Decreased level of consciousness
- Pauses in breathing
- Decreased urine volume
- Murmuring to people others cannot see
- Reaching in air or picking at covers
- Need for assistance with all care

Days to Hours Before Passing

- Decreased level of consciousness or comatoselike state
- Inability to swallow
- Pauses in breathing become longer
- Shallow breaths
- Knees, feet, and/or hands becoming cool or cold
- Knees, feet, and/or hands discoloring to purplish hue
- Skin coloring becoming pale, waxen

❧ WILL I BE ALONE? ❧

Will Others Be with You in Your Final Days or Hours?

Thomas and Luanne

"I JUST DON'T KNOW WHAT TO DO," Luanne says, wrapping her knobby, arthritic fingers around her coffee mug as we sit together at her kitchen table. "He won't stay in bed. We've tried keeping the rails up, but he just climbs over them. Our daughter tries to help, but she just had hip surgery. I want to keep him at home, but I don't know if I can. If he won't stay in bed, if he keeps falling . . ."

Thomas, Luanne's husband, is ninety-three years old. He and Luanne have been married for seventy-two years. They live in the country, in the same house they've shared since their daughter was born.

"Are you sure I can't get you a cup of coffee?" she asks.

I smile and shake my head. "Thank you, but no, I'm fine. I suspect you're pretty tired."

She nods. "I am, but we promised each other we'd do our best to keep the other one at home, right to the end. I'm trying, but . . ."

I lay a gentle hand on her arm. "You're doing an amazing job."

"Thank you . . . I don't get much sleep. He's so restless. He talks. His arms move all around, and then he tries to crawl out of the bed. I do my best to keep him safe, but . . ."

"Can you understand what he's saying?"

"He just keeps saying he has to go. I ask if he has to go to the bathroom, and it's as if he doesn't even hear me. I don't think that's the problem, though. We've been using the disposable underwear for a couple of weeks now. It doesn't seem to bother him. He doesn't even know when he's—" She catches her words, as if embarrassed for him.

"That's okay. It happens." I gaze at this extraordinary woman, at the strength that lies within her small, bent frame. What stories could she tell if we had more time? What will her life be like when the house is empty, when she, perhaps for the first time in her life, is alone?

"Shall we go see him?" I ask.

We enter the room and find Thomas on his knees, attempting to crawl over the rails of the bed. He's small, bony, frail. Loose skin droops from arms where once there had been muscle. He'd been a farmer. He and Luanne worked the land and raised a daughter here. Fifteen years ago, in the face of urban sprawl and advancing age, they sold much of the land, keeping only a few acres around the house.

I approach the bed. Thomas doesn't look at me. Instead, he leans to one side, to see around me, focused on something behind me. "Thomas," I say gently. He makes no response. I step closer. Then I take another step, this time moving very close.

I look to his eyes for some recognition of my presence. But I see none. Instead, he leans right, around me, still intent on the space beyond me. Staying close, I lean right. He then leans left. I lean left. We continue like this for some time—he still looking beyond me, around me, not seeing me, I moving with him, remaining close.

Finally, he stops. His brows furrow, and for the first time since I arrived in the room, he sees me.

"Thomas, your wife is here with me. We cannot see what you see. Can you tell us what you see?"

He stares at me for a moment. Then once more he looks around me. His frail arm lifts to point. "There's a river. It's sparkling. It's so bright, the sunlight . . . it's so bright . . . And there, on the other side of the river, Tim and Al, Tony and Nate are waiting. There's a boat. I have to get in it. I have to go to them. They're waiting for me. I have to go . . . It's beautiful . . . It's beautiful . . . It's so beautiful . . ."

Still gazing at the place only he can see, he resumes his attempts to get out of the bed. I turn to Luanne.

Tears flow down her face. "Those are his brothers . . . They're all gone now. He's the last one."

Epilogue

Luanne and her daughter decide to lightly sedate Thomas to keep him safe, to prevent him from falling. Though he's no longer able to get out of bed, he's still conscious, still able to murmur, still able to reach in the air until he passes away, two days later, at home, with Luanne at his side.

*There is a great difference between still believing something,
and believing it again.*

— Georg Christoph Lichtenberg

We are here to awaken from the illusion of our separateness.

—Thich Nhat Hanh

COMMON EXPERIENCES OF THOSE NEARING DEATH

People are often only minimally aware of what is occurring around them, but appear to be participating in events others cannot see.

Some common behaviors include:

- Fingers plucking at the covers
- Reaching or grasping at objects not seen by others
- Seeing people others cannot see
- Asking for loved ones who are deceased
- Seeing and/or talking with loved ones who are deceased
- Stating "I need to go" or using similar language, often accompanied by restlessness
- Attempting to go toward what they see

To learn more about near death awareness and experience, read *Consciousness Beyond Life: The Science of the Near-Death Experience* by Pim van Lommel.

❧ WILL I CHOOSE MY TIME? ❧

Does the Mind or Spirit Influence When We Pass?

Pete

"I've been waiting for you," Pete says, wheeling his chair toward me as I step in the door to start my shift at the hospice. "I've decided I'm ready to go today."

"Go where?" I ask, surprised to see Pete up at 6:30 in the morning.

"I've decided that I've taken care of everything I need to. I've fought long and hard. I'm ready to let go and pass on to whatever's next. I've decided to die today."

I sit beside him. He's on more than a dozen medications and artificial IV nutrition—aggressive therapy designed to prolong life. "Today?"

Pete nods. "Today."

"Okay," I say, keeping my skepticism concealed. Even if we stop the medications and IV nutrition, he likely won't pass for at least another week. But this is his life, and I'm here to support him.

"Can we talk in the garden?" he asks.

I follow as he wheels out the door and down the path, into a patch of early morning sunshine. "Did something happen to bring you to this decision?" I ask.

He squints at the sun. Finally, he shakes his head. "You know, I'm just ready. I've made my peace with this, with a lot of other things in my life—the good and the bad. I have a lot of good friends, and I'll miss them, but it's time." He turns to me. "It's not so much about being tired of this life, this fight. Yeah, it's pretty tough a lot of the time. But I guess I've reached a place where I accept that I've finished all I need to, and I'm ready to discover whatever's next."

His mouth lifts in a crooked smile. "You know, I never imagined I'd be at this point. It just kind of happened. And it's like this huge weight

9

has lifted off me. Call it acceptance; call it peace; call it whatever you like," he shrugs. "But the sun is shining, and I feel good about this. I'm ready to let go and let whatever happens, happen."

"How can we support you?"

He reaches for my hands. "Thank you." He draws a deep breath. "I've been sitting out here, watching the sun come up, thinking about what I want today. I think I'd like peaceful things around me. I'd like to spend the morning in the garden. I'd also like a big breakfast of eggs and bacon and pancakes. I probably can't eat it, but I can taste it, a bite or two maybe, and I'd enjoy that.

"After breakfast I'd like to come back to the garden and plant a rosebush. A friend of mine has been keeping my roses for me since I got sick. I used to keep a few bushes on my apartment patio. They're really beautiful, with this abundance of soft, pink, delicate blooms that smell wonderful. Whenever the first buds appeared I knew that summer was just around the corner."

He smiles. "I'd like to leave something here for the people who come after me. Something to make them smile. Something that will remind them, even with all they have to deal with, that there are still wonderful things, like blooming roses, all around them."

"Thank you. That's a nice gift to give everyone."

"In the afternoon I'd like to have a few friends come by for a visit. I don't think I want to tell them I'm going today. I just want to enjoy being with them. I want to laugh with them. I want to have a good time. Maybe they can help me plant the rosebush.

"Then in the early evening I'd like a long, hot bath in the Jacuzzi tub, with scented soap." He turns to the garden. "I've lost most of my sense of taste, but my sense of smell is still keen. It's something I still enjoy."

He gazes at the garden for a few moments. "Afterward I'd like a massage with some scented candles burning. I'd like some nice music, too. Mozart, maybe. Then I think I'll just close my eyes and let go."

"Okay," I say. "I'll get breakfast ordered and arrange for the massage. I'll also make sure the rest of the staff know what you want."

He reaches for my hand and gives it a firm squeeze. "No more medicine. No more IVs."

I nod. "No more."

At the end of my shift I step into the garden and join Pete as he sits beside his rosebush, helping it settle into its new home. Seeing me approach, he snips a delicate bloom. "Here," he says, offering it to me. "Enjoy."

I reach for the blossom. "Thank you," I say quietly, wondering if I should say good-bye, wondering how he will feel if he doesn't pass as he plans, when he has more days, a week, longer perhaps, to wait for his body to catch up with his spirit on the next step of his journey.

He takes me in his arms. "Let's not say good-bye," he whispers. Then he straightens. He manages a smile and a small wave.

I take my cue. We exchange one last, meaningful smile that speaks a language of its own. Then I turn to leave.

The next morning I pull into the parking lot, thinking about Pete, hoping he can still feel that sense of peace, not disappointment, or anger, or frustration at not passing as he planned. I step in the door and am astounded. Just before midnight, as the scent of lavender filled the air and Mozart played, Pete passed away.

Hal and Jane

Late in the night at the hospice house, I assess Hal. He is nonresponsive. His body tells me he will live another few days.

Jane, his wife, draws his hand to her tear-stained cheek. "I just want to be with him . . ." They are newlyweds, she tells me. Both in their late forties, neither had expected to find such a deep love.

She then shares the rest of the story, of his visit to the doctor the week before for a persistent headache. The headache hadn't stopped him from working, or exercising at the gym, or biking. The news came two days later: an inoperable brain tumor.

Anticipating a lifetime to share a love she never expected to find, she is devastated. Hal is strangely accepting of the situation. He exhibits no denial, no anger, no fear. He supports her as best he can, but tells her, "I'm ready. I accept this. I'm at peace. I hope you'll find peace as well."

I look at the man who only a week before was fully engaged in life, who only moments ago I believed would live another few days. Physically, his body is not yet at that edge, but I realize it's his spirit, his sense of peace and acceptance that leads the way. "Would you like to spend the night in the bed with him?" I ask.

Jane looks up. "Can I?"

In the first light of morning, lying in Jane's arms, Hal takes his final breaths.

The only journey is the journey within.
—Rainer Maria Rilke

Suggestions for Achieving Acceptance

Why are you ready to let go?

- ✦ Do you wish for your life to end as quickly as possible, or are you at peace and open to whatever may come?
- ✦ If you wish for your life to end quickly, why? Can the reasons for your unhappiness as you experience this remaining time be addressed or resolved?

See "I'm Afraid to Lose Control . . ." (page 124), "I'm Not Ready . . ." (page 131), "Is It Too Late to Make Amends?" (page 137), and "I'm Ready—Why Am I Not Going?" (page 141).

To achieve peace with your situation and acceptance of what may come, consider the following:

- ✦ Conclude any unfinished business.
- ✦ Surround yourself with what holds meaning and offers peace to you.
- ✦ Say good-bye to loved ones.
- ✦ Feel no pressure to adhere to a time line or schedule.
- ✦ Accept and enjoy the passage of time, whether hours, days, or weeks, until you pass.

❋ WILL I BE AWARE? ❋

The Possibility of Consciousness, Even If We're Not Awake or Responsive

Jim

"JIM," I WHISPER, LEANING CLOSE TO THE unresponsive man in the bed in the hospice house. "I'm still trying to reach your wife. There's no answer. But I'll keep trying."

"Do you think he can hear you, that he understands?" asks Jim's fifty-year-old son, Michael, as he sits beside his father, gently holding his hand.

I nod. "My colleagues and I could tell you hundreds of stories of people like your father, who are not responsive and are very close to passing, who show us, in some small way, that they understand."

"Really?"

Again I nod. "Last week we cared for a young man whose mother lived in Chicago and couldn't be here. For two days he hadn't made any response, even when we gently turned him every couple of hours. When he was close to passing, we called his mother and held the phone to his ear. As she spoke, we watched these subtle facial expressions form, a slight movement of his mouth, eyelids fluttering, things like that. After the call, he again became completely unresponsive, and remained that way until he died an hour later.

"So even when people can't respond," I add, "when they appear comatose, we talk to them. We tell them what we're about to do so they're not startled by our touch. We tell them who we've talked to, who's coming in, and when they'll be here. The rest is up to them."

"What do you mean?"

"Over the years I've come to believe that, to some extent, we choose our time to pass. Some people wait for a loved one to arrive. Others pass when they're alone, as if to spare their loved one from witnessing that final moment of life, or to experience that transition privately. For each person, that moment of departure seems like the perfect choice, given his unique situation. But choice requires awareness. How that awareness occurs, I don't know. I just see it happen, over and over. So I accept the possibility, and act with that belief.

"If he can hear me, he knows what's happening. If he can't . . ." I shrug. "Then I'm just talking and it doesn't matter. But I'd rather give him the benefit of the doubt."

Michael gazes at his father. "I see what you mean."

"So if there are things you want to say to him, maybe in some way, he can hear you."

Michael gazes at his father, then gently smoothes a stray lock of his hair. "I'll leave you two," I say, stepping toward the door. "I'll keep trying to reach his wife."

Twenty minutes later I return. I lean close to Jim. "I just reached Madeleine. She'll be here in half an hour." I hesitate. Should I tell him the rest? "I'll come," she'd said. "But I will not go into that room. I can't bear to see him like that."

Madeleine cannot bear to see him. And she cannot bear to see his son.

Michael and Jim met only recently. One day Michael's mother, Connie, showed him a faded photograph of a young man in uniform, taken in the troubled days of World War II. "That's your father," she'd said. "I should have told you long ago."

Michael made contact with Jim. Jim was stunned and overjoyed. But Madeleine, Jim's wife of forty-six years, a stern, deeply devout woman, was horrified. Unable to have children of her own, she refused to acknowledge Michael's existence. She didn't allow him in her house, and refused to even look at him.

Despite this, Jim and Michael forged a bond. What began as cautious talks over coffee evolved into mornings with fishing poles at a river's edge, the hours passing without the need for conversation.

When Jim became ill and was frequently hospitalized, finding time together became increasingly difficult. But somehow they managed to share moments together while honoring Madeleine's wishes, allowing her never to find Michael at Jim's side or near his room.

Michael wipes tears from his cheeks. "I should go now."

"You have a little time," I offer gently. "It will take her about a half-hour to arrive."

Michael gazes at his father. "I'll stay just a little longer. But I'll leave before she gets here. I wish I could stay. I wish I could be with him, but I can't make this any more difficult for her than it already is."

"I'll leave you to share your last moments together." Silently, I wish Jim peace, knowing the impossible position he's in—the two people he loves the most cannot be together with him. The son who loves him, who wants to be with him, must go. The wife who loves him, but cannot bear to see him as he dies, will arrive.

As I turn to leave, I hear Jim's breathing change. I look back, startled, watching as Jim's chin and throat lift, as his jaw lowers then closes, the characteristic final breaths.

"Michael . . ."

Michael looks up.

"Your father is taking his last breaths." I step out and gently close the door.

Moments later Michael opens the door. "He's gone."

I gather him into my arms as the tears flow anew.

"I'm so glad," he says at last, his voice muffled against my shoulder. "I'm so glad I got to know him. And I'm so glad I could be here with him. I wish Madeleine . . . I'm sorry she didn't make it in time."

He straightens and wipes his eyes. "I should go . . . I don't want to, not yet, but . . ."

"We have a little time before Madeline arrives." I share how we honor people at their passing, by washing and dressing their body, then placing a special quilt, what we call a passage quilt, over them, folded beneath their arms like a light blanket, always leaving their face, arms, and hands uncovered. I tell him that some families choose to participate, or to gather after, while some do not. It's up to him to stay or to go.

He gazes at his father. "Is there time for me to do that for him? I want to, but . . . I need to honor Madeleine, too."

"I'll keep a close eye on the time," I promise. So together we bathe Jim, and Michael chooses the quilt. In its colors are the mixed hues of a river in sunlight, of life beneath the surface, seen but not seen, a universe in flow, splashing, moving, changing.

After we place the quilt, Michael steps back and smiles at his father. "He looks good for her." He gives me one last hug. "I'm so glad I could be here with him."

I notice his trembling hands. "Would you like to wait in another part of the building? Maybe take a moment to reflect before you drive home?"

He considers my question, then nods. "That's probably a good idea."

I lead him to the other end of the building, to a quiet room families often use for reflection or prayer. I return to find Madeleine entering the building, accompanied by a friend. Her movements are abrupt, tense. I take her hands in mine and gently tell her that Jim has passed.

She stares at me, then draws her hands away. "I don't want to see him."

I nod. "That's okay. Whatever is right for you."

She turns to leave.

"We have some of his things," I say to her retreating back. "His watch, his pajamas . . ."

She turns slightly, frowning. "Keep them. I don't want them. I donate them to the hospice." She steps out the door and is gone.

I find Michael sitting alone in the dark. Without a word I hand him his father's watch. He stares at it. Tears well up in his eyes. He slips it on his wrist.

It just ain't possible to explain some things. It's interesting to wonder on them and do some speculation, but the main thing is you have to accept it—and get on with your growing.

—Jim Dodge

Sharing Time with Your Unresponsive Loved One

- Assume that your loved one may be aware of your presence and can hear you.
- Share your feelings as you wish to.
- If you are providing physical care, tell the person what you will do before you begin, and continue to inform her prior to each touch or action throughout the process.
- As you sit with your loved one, consider using this time for quiet reflection or prayer, reading, journaling, or some other calming activity.
- If you wish to talk, consider reminiscing about shared experiences, acknowledging lessons learned, attributes admired, difficult experiences, and wisdom gained.
- Tell your loved one when you are leaving, and when you'll return.
- When you leave, accept that this may be the last time you see your loved one. Depart feeling as if you've said all you wish to say.
- For information on signs of approaching death, see "How Will We Know When the End Is Near?" (page 170).
- For information about creating a peaceful environment near the time of death, see "I Want to Be with Her When She Passes . . ." (page 179).
- For information on verbalizations or gestures people often make near the time of death, see "Will I Be Alone?" (page 6).

❈ I HAD THIS DREAM... ❈
A Description of Common Dream Themes

Nguyen, Two Months before His Passing

"HE'S BEEN HAVING THESE VIVID DREAMS," Mai says about her father, Nguyen. "He says he knows they must be dreams, but they seem very real."

"Are you frightened by them?" I ask Nguyen, trying to determine if it's a medication hallucination—a hallucination of frightening objects—or the vivid, but not frightening dreams that commonly occur during the end-of-life journey.

Mai translates my question and Nguyen shakes his head.

"What do you dream about?" I ask.

Mai translates and the creases of Nguyen's leathered face deepen into a smile.

"He says in his dreams his old friends come to visit him, friends he has not seen since we left Vietnam many, many years ago. He says everyone is old now, like him. They sit together in the courtyard of our house in Huê, like it used to be, before the war. They play *Tiên Lên* and drink lotus tea and tell each other stories about what has happened in their lives since they were last together."

Nguyen begins speaking again, his hands moving in their own animated translation.

"He says he is very happy to see them. He says he has wondered many times over the years what has happened to them."

Again Nguyen speaks. Mai listens, then turns to me. "He wants to know what the dreams mean."

"I don't know what they mean. But I can tell you that it's fairly common to have vivid dreams like this, beginning a few months prior to our passing.

"Right now your dreams are about seeing your old friends. Later the theme of the dreams may change. You may dream that you're waiting to take a trip, or that you've begun the trip and can glimpse what's ahead, but can't get there yet. Later, people often dream of water. Some people dream of saying good-bye. Most people report these dreams to be peaceful, happy experiences."

Mai translates. Then Nguyen smiles at me. Mai translates his words.

"He says he is very, very happy to see his old friends again . . ."

Sandra, a Few Weeks before Her Passing

"I'm having trouble sleeping," Sandra shares. "It's not that I don't sleep. I just wake up restless, feeling as if I haven't slept. I have these dreams. They wake me up. It's like I have to go somewhere."

"What do you dream about?" I ask.

"Well, last night I dreamt that a coach, like an old stagecoach, was waiting outside my window. The other night it was a train. It's as if I have to go somewhere. The coach is there, but I'm not ready to get in . . ."

Fred, a Week before Passing

"I think I'm hallucinating," Fred says, waking up from a nap.

I kneel beside his bed. "What do you see?"

He scratches his head. "I don't know if I see it, or if it's a dream. It's as if I'm on an island, surrounded by water."

"Are you frightened?"

Vigorously he shakes his head. "No. Not at all." Then his gaze wanders beyond me. He smiles. "It's serene . . . It's beautiful . . . It's so beautiful. I've never known such peace."

Wayne, Two Days before Passing

"Oh, you startled me!" Beth, my colleague says to Wayne as he grips her hand. Wayne has been drifting in and out of consciousness for the last six days. A moment ago he'd been lying unconscious in the bed. And then, with eyes still closed, he reached for Beth's hand as she bent to check on him.

"I went looking for you," he whispers in a weak voice. "Why did you go down there?"

Beth's brows wrinkle. "Down where?"

"To that room, a little room, with lots of windows, with sunlight streaming in . . ."

Beth's eyes widen. Wayne has not left his room since he arrived at the hospice house a week before. He's seen only the entrance to the building and the hallway leading to his room. He could not possibly have known of the rooms at the far end of the building, nor could he have known that Beth had just taken a short lunch break, not in the staff room where she usually goes, but at the far end of the building, far beyond the patient rooms, in the Sun Room, a little room with lots of windows, with sunlight streaming in . . .

"You looked happy to be there," Wayne whispers.

The most beautiful thing we can experience is the mysterious.

—*Albert Einstein*

COMMON DREAM THEMES

Vivid dreams often begin occurring months to weeks before passing, and occur during sleep. Most people who experience them wake up and are able to recall some of the dream.

Common dream themes include:

Dreams of closure: May include seeing old friends or family, both living and deceased.

Dreams of a pending trip: May include a feeling of restlessness, of waiting, but not yet being able to depart.

Dreams of a body of water: Frequently, the dreamer is on one side of the water and wishes to cross, but cannot. This is often described as being beautiful, peaceful, or serene.

Though rare, some people have out-of-body experiences and may be able to relate a visual or auditory experience they could not otherwise have witnessed.

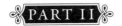

❧ PART II ❧

What Will Happen? The Physical Journey

This section offers information that may be helpful to individuals coping with declining health.

In this section you'll learn what this journey may be like for you. You'll learn what physical and emotional changes you may experience, and discover tools to cope with these changes. You'll also learn about some of the legal and practical issues you and your loved ones may face, and ways to address them. Most chapters are followed by a list of suggestions, tools, or other resources to help you develop a solution that reflects your unique needs and values.

What Should I Do Now?
Expressing Your Wishes
How to Complete Advance Directive and Medical Power of Attorney
Forms

Will I Be in Pain?
How Pain Medication Works
When to Use It
What to Tell Your Doctor
How to Minimize Side Effects
Understanding Common Pain Medication Myths

I Don't Want to Be a Burden . . .
Ways to View and Cope with Dependence

I Wish I Had More Energy . . .
Tools to Maximize Energy and Mobility

Do I Want to Help Plan My Remembrance Service?
Ways to Explore This Topic with Loved Ones

❋ What Should I Do Now? ❋

Expressing Your Wishes
How to Complete Advance Directive and
Medical Power of Attorney Forms

Pauline and Benjamin

"She must have signed in the wrong place . . ." Benjamin's voice trails off as he stares at the advance directive that Pauline, his wife, has signed. His hand trembles as he holds the paper. "I'm sure she didn't mean that . . ."

I swallow. In the adjacent room, Pauline lies in a vegetative state, kept alive by a feeding tube, with no conscious volition. She receives meticulous care from Dimitra, the gracious woman who runs the adult foster home where she now lives.

Pauline is unaware that Benjamin, her husband of fifty-three years, who still enjoys an active life playing tennis and golf, chose to move into the small bedroom at the adult foster home simply to be with her, to hear her breathe, to hold her limp hand, to bend down and brush his lips against hers, wishing her good morning, good night.

Benjamin, shaking his head, sets down the advance directive. "She must have signed in the wrong place," he rasps. Then biting his lip, he turns away.

I wait. Five years ago, Pauline talked with her doctor about the fate that might await her. Afterward, she completed an advance directive. One by one she answered the difficult questions of what she would want if she were no longer able to communicate in any way, no longer able to live without the support of medical interventions like feeding tubes or breathing machines, no longer able to recognize her family, and no possibility of recovery existed.

Using the form, Pauline clearly indicated that she did not want life-extending treatment. "I DO NOT want tube feeding. I DO NOT want resuscitation . . ." At the end of the document she wrote, in her own hand, "I do not want my life to be prolonged by life support."

But Benjamin cannot see this. I gaze at him as he stares out the window, at Dimitra's young children as they play in the yard. How great the burden must be to let go of someone you love, of someone with whom you've shared a lifetime. How great the burden to choose a course that will bring an end to the breathing you listen to each night as you fall asleep, to know that if you follow this course, you will be alone.

I think about Pauline. How great the burden must have been to make these choices. What courage she must have found to look deep within her soul to choose what life, what living, meant to her. Was a heartbeat enough? Was it enough simply to breathe? For her, what did it mean, truly, to be alive?

Benjamin reaches for my hand. Without looking at me he says, "I can't let her go."

"I know," I whisper. Finally, I say, "She's a very lucky woman to share life with someone who loves her so much."

Benjamin shakes his head. "I was the lucky one . . ."

We sit together quietly, neither saying a word, Benjamin holding my hand.

"I suppose you think I should let her go," he says at last.

I shake my head. "This isn't about what I think. It's about what Pauline thinks, what she would want."

Benjamin expels a shaking breath and tears roll down his cheeks. "I can't make that choice." He lets go of my hand and wipes his tear-stained face.

"She's not asking you to." I wrap my arm around his shaking shoulders. "She loved you enough not to put you in the position to have to choose."

He stares at me, his brow wrinkling in confusion.

"She didn't want to ask that of you. She knew it would be an impossible choice. Instead, *she* made the choice. She wrote it down. And she had it witnessed. She did this, she chose, so you wouldn't have to decide what living meant to her.

"Through this document she said that when she reached this point, when she no longer knew you, when she no longer knew her children, her grandchildren, when she could no longer interact with anyone, she said, 'That isn't living—not to me. Don't hook me up to machines. Don't keep me alive. Let me go.'"

Tears continue to stream down Benjamin's face. He turns to the advance directive. Slowly, he picks it up and reads again, one by one, the questions, and Pauline's answers.

How we spend our days is, of course, how we spend our lives.
—Annie Dillard

ENSURING THAT YOUR WISHES ARE HONORED
To ensure that your choices are honored, consider taking the following actions:

- Examine your values about life and living.
- Communicate your values to your loved ones, and specify your wishes in writing, using an Advance Directive form.
- Select a person to make medical decisions for you if you become unable to make decisions for yourself. Communicate your choices and values to this person to ensure that she'll make decisions that reflect your values. You will use a Medical Power of Attorney form to officially designate this person as you health care decision maker or proxy.
- Ask your health care provider for Advance Directive and Medical Power of Attorney forms. U.S. residents can also obtain their state's forms online at no cost. For more information, see "Appendix A: Additional Resources" (page 210).
- If you have completed Advance Directive and Medical Power of Attorney forms in one state or province, but have since moved to a different state or province, you must complete new forms for your current state or province.
- Carefully follow the directions provided, including requirements

for having your signature witnessed. U.S. residents do not need an attorney to help complete Advance Directive and Medical Power of Attorney forms. Residents of other countries should consult their health care provider regarding applicable rules and laws.

* Give copies to your health care decision maker and to your health care provider. If you have hospice care, provide copies to your hospice team as well.

* If you have chosen not to be resuscitated, ask your health care provider for a Do Not Resuscitate (DNR) order to place in your home. In many U.S. states, if paramedics are called to a home and find a person without a heartbeat, they must, by law, attempt resuscitation unless a valid DNR order is available. Even if you have completed an advance directive and state that you do not want resuscitation, you must also obtain a DNR order. An advance directive, while a statement of your wishes, is not a legally binding medical order. A DNR order is. (In some states, this form is called a POLST: Physician's Order for Life Sustaining Treatment.)

* If you do obtain a DNR order, consider taping it to your refrigerator or another location where it can be easily located in an emergency.

* For more information about medical issues, such as resuscitation and artificial nutrition, read *Hard Choices for Loving People* by Hank Dunn. For information about how to locate a copy of this booklet, see "Appendix A: Additional Resources" (page 210).

* Investigate the need for a property will for distribution of your assets. For suggested resources for estate planning, see "Appendix A: Additional Resources" (page 210).

* Put together in one place all your important documents, such as your birth certificate, your insurance papers, your marriage certificate, and the like. See "Appendix B: Important Documents to Gather" (page 215).

* If you have a pet, will your loved ones continue to care for it after you pass? If not, ask your loved ones for help finding a good home for it after you pass.

❋ WILL I BE IN PAIN? ❋

How Pain Medication Works
When to Use It
What to Tell Your Doctor
How to Minimize Side Effects
Understanding Common Pain Medication Myths

Sam and Margaret

SAM SITS HUNCHED IN HIS ARMCHAIR IN the house where he and Margaret have lived for forty-eight years. Pictures of pigtailed granddaughters, a wedding party, and a young man in uniform share space on the end table with a hand-carved wooden owl Sam made in his woodshop. The deep lines worn in his leather belt show just how much weight he's lost in the last six months. The deep lines on his face show the pain he tries to hide.

"I don't want to take any of that," he says of the bottle of Vicodin that sits unused on the kitchen counter. "I'll keep taking Tylenol."

Margaret comes around the corner with a basket of freshly washed laundry. "I've tried to tell him to take it—that he'll feel better—but he won't." She sits on the couch and starts to fold towels. "I think he's afraid that if he takes it now, it won't work later, if things get worse. But I can tell; he hurts all the time."

"I don't want to be some kind of addict," Sam says. "And I don't want to feel drugged." He shakes his head. "I can get through it."

Margaret frowns. "I know you don't want to admit it, but . . . Please, Sam." She pushes the laundry aside and places a loving hand on Sam's knee. "I've seen you try to hide it. I've seen you wince when you move. You don't think I see it, but I do, and—" Her voice catches. "I hate to see you in pain. I know you don't want to take that medicine, but maybe we can find something that will work . . ."

I gaze at Sam, who turns away. "This must be hard for you, for both of you," I say.

Still looking away, Sam slowly nods.

It's Okay to Admit That You Hurt

For many people, admitting we feel pain is as if we're admitting defeat. "If only I were stronger, if I could just tough it out . . ." Sometimes it feels as if admitting to pain and taking medication are signs of weakness, that if we admit to pain, the disease somehow wins.

What pain does is consume our energy. It makes us restless. It can rob us of our appetite. It can make us irritable.

You can continue to be stoic, Sam, to choose not to take medicine, but it's likely that the pain will consume a significant amount of your energy. You probably won't want to visit with people. You'll probably withdraw because you hurt. When your children and grandchildren come to visit, you'll be spending most of your energy trying to not let them see that you're in pain.

No one but you can decide what's most important to you, what the right choices are. Your body is dealing with this disease. You've fought long and hard. With this disease, most people feel some pain. It's not weakness. It's not giving in. It's the disease.

So the choice is this: Do you take control of the pain? And if so, what will work best for you

I Don't Want to Get Addicted, and I Don't Want to Feel Drugged

Let's start with your concern about addiction. When we experience harm, our body transmits signals to get our attention. Pain medicine works by matching up with the receptors in our brain and spine that receive these signals. It's as if the pain medication steps between the signals of pain and the places in the brain and spine that receive these signals, blocking them.

Now, if we're not experiencing harm and our body isn't making those signals, if we don't have pain, when the pain medicine matches with the receptors, there's nothing to consume the pain medication—no signal to block. So instead, the chemicals of the medicine, specifically narcotic pain medications, send a different message, one of altered perception, elation, or even euphoria. That's what creates addiction—the craving for that altered perception, that euphoria.

But you have pain, Sam. Your body is sending those signals. So the pain medicine will be absorbed the way it's intended to and will do its job. You should be as clear in your thinking with the pain medicine as you are now without it. Over the years I've worked with hundreds of people taking high doses of pain medication with no alteration in their thinking.

WHAT ABOUT SIDE EFFECTS?

When you first start taking narcotic pain medication, you might feel some side effects as your body adjusts. In most people, these side effects resolve in forty-eight to seventy-two hours. You might feel nausea. You might also sleep a little more than usual, or feel groggy, or foggy. Because of that, you'll want to be a little more cautious when you first get up and begin to move around. But, again, these side effects should last only a day or two, three at the most. So if you have these side effects, give the medicine a few days before you give up on it. Chances are your body will adapt. If it doesn't, we'll try something else.

In some very rare cases, some people are actually allergic to the medicine. If you develop a rash, or swelling of your tongue, or shortness of breath, call hospice immediately.

The side effect of narcotic pain meds that, unfortunately, won't go away is constipation. You'll need to take a laxative, and we pesky nurses are going to ask you, every time we visit, when you've had a bowel movement. If you get behind and don't have a bowel movement at least every two or three days, you'll need to increase the laxatives. We're sorry to be so nosy about your bowel movements, but we don't want you to feel relief from the pain but experience an entirely different, preventable pain from constipation.

A good way to keep track is to keep a calendar in the bathroom. Just mark the days when you have a bowel movement. Using that record, the health care team will work with you to find the right balance of laxatives and stool softeners.

How to Know How Much Pain Medication You Need

You'll want to keep track of when you take the medicine, how much you take, and if it helps. Write this in a notebook, and keep the notebook handy.

You'll probably start with a short-acting pain medicine. Short-acting medicines are not timed-release. That means that once you take it, you should start feeling some relief in about thirty minutes. You'll feel the full effect of the medicine in about an hour, and it will last in your system and continue to work for about three to four hours.

Often, doctors will prescribe a range of medicine to allow you some flexibility. For this medicine, your doctor prescribed one-half to two tablets every four hours, as needed for pain. The best approach would be to start with the smallest amount, in this case, a half-tablet. If you're still in pain after the medicine has reached its peak, in one hour, take another half-tablet. See if that works. If not, take more. Just don't exceed what the doctor has prescribed, in this case, two tablets in four hours. If you're still not comfortable, call hospice. We need to know. We'll call your doctor to get the right dose, or maybe try a different medicine.

The next time you feel pain, get out your notebook. Ask yourself if this pain feels as strong as it did the last time. If so, look back to see how much pain medicine you needed. If you needed one-and-a-half tablets to get comfortable, then chances are you'll need one-and-a-half tablets this time, too. Or if the pain isn't as strong, or you're not sure, take a little less, and see if you need more.

Also, you might feel relief initially, but the pain may come back again before the four hours are up. If that happens, check your notebook to see how much you've taken in the last four hours. Add it up. If the total is less than the largest dose the doctor has prescribed, then you can take more, up to that amount.

After four hours, the short-acting medicine will be out of your system, so it's as if you're starting over. You add up only what's been taken of the short-acting medicine in the time frame the doctor prescribes.

If you find that you need to take pain medicine regularly, more than three or four times a day, we'll add a long-acting, timed-release medicine. The advantage of a long-acting medicine is that you don't have to wait for the medicine to go to work, and you don't have to worry about it wearing off. You can sleep for several hours and not wake up in pain. Since long-acting medicine is released slowly in your system, you'll still need the short-acting medicine for those times when you're more active, or if something else triggers some additional pain.

That's another reason why keeping track is important. It will help us work together to determine the amount of medicine you need, and the right schedule for you.

The other thing to keep in mind is *when* to take pain medication. Once you start to feel pain, the longer you wait before you take the pain medication, the more medicine you'll need to get the pain under control. So you might wait, thinking that it will get better, but instead your body simply sends more and more pain signals. So if you wait, chances are you'll need more medicine to get it under control.

Different Types of Pain Call for Different Types of Medicine

Pain has different causes, and based on its cause, there are differences in how it feels. For example, it may feel like pressure, or a sharp stab, or a burning sensation, or something else. It's important for us to know what it feels like, because for each cause, there are different medicines. We'll want to match the right medicine to the cause of pain.

In some people, there might be more than one cause, so if something about your pain changes—the character, the location, or its intensity—let us know and we'll work with your doctor to choose the right medicines.

Sometimes what causes or worsens pain isn't always physical. The end-of-life process brings up many emotional and spiritual issues.

Sometimes these issues can create anxiety or tension. If these issues aren't addressed and resolved, then that anxiety or tension can increase to a point where it develops into real, physical pain.

Earlier, I mentioned working with a team. That team includes the physician, nurses, social workers, pharmacists, nurse's aides, volunteers, and, if you choose, chaplains. It takes all of us to help a person, a family, achieve true comfort.

WHAT IF THE MEDICINE DOESN'T WORK? WILL I BE IN PAIN?

With good communication with the health care team, most people—no matter what their disease—are able to achieve physical comfort without any sedation or grogginess caused by pain medication. In addition to medicines, we use a lot of other tools, things like hot or cold packs, massage, guided imagery, even spiritual support. It's *very* rare that we can't get someone comfortable using conventional approaches. But if that does happen—and, again, it's rare—we still have options. We *can* make you comfortable.

Everyone is unique. What might work well for one person, might not work for another. Ultimately, you're in charge. You make the choices. You tell us what you want, what's working, what's not working, and we'll find the right medicines, the right doses, the right tools, the right support for you.

You gain strength, courage, and confidence by every experience in which you really stop to look fear in the face.

—Eleanor Roosevelt

MANAGING PAIN MEDICATION

- ✦ Talk with your doctor, pharmacist, or nurse to understand how your medication works.
- ✦ Be sure to understand how long each medication lasts, if it's short-acting, or timed-release.

- If the medication is timed-release, swallow it whole. Do not chew or dissolve it in your mouth.
- Understand the dosage. Is it prescribed as a single dose, or is there a range? (For example, "Take one to two tablets every four hours, as needed for pain.")
- Understand how often the medication can be taken. (Let's use the same example: "Take one to two tablets every four hours, as needed for pain." Let's say you experience pain at noon and take one tablet. At one o'clock, you still feel some pain and take a second tablet. By one-thirty you feel much better, but at four-thirty the pain returns. Since you can take the medication every four hours, using your log, add up what you've taken in the last four hours—in this case, one tablet three and a half hours ago, at one o'clock. Since you can take up to two tablets in four hours, you can take another tablet now, and, if you need it, a second tablet after five o'clock.)
- Ask if there's a limit to how much can be taken in twenty-four hours.
- Ask your health care provider for help in finding the right dose of laxatives and stool softeners for you.
- Keep a record of how much of each medicine you take, when you take it, and if it's effective. Share it with your health care provider.
- Tell your health care provider if your pain changes in any way.
- If you need more than three or four doses of short-acting pain medication each day, talk with your health care provider about adding or increasing the dose of a timed-release medication.
- To prevent constipation, keep a record of your bowel movements. If you've not had a bowel movement in three days (or if you begin to experience loose bowel movements) call your health care provider and ask for help in adjusting your laxative dose.
- For more information about common pain medications, see "Appendix C: Common Pain Medications" (page 216).
- For more information about other ways to improve comfort, see "Appendix D: Supportive Therapies" (page 218).

I Don't Want to Be a Burden . . .

Ways to View and Cope with Dependence

Meredith and Her Daughters

"Let me help you," Ginny says, hurrying toward her mom, Meredith, who is struggling to rise from the recliner in her living room.

I set down my bag and take a step toward them to help. Then, seeing Ginny's care and competency, I step back.

"No, I can do it," Meredith insists as she struggles. "Just let me do this. I don't need help."

Ginny stands beside her mom, her feet braced slightly apart. A few steps away, Kathy and Melinda, Meredith's other daughters, are also poised to help. We wait, watching Meredith, giving her the chance to do what she's able to, what she wants to do.

"I can do this," Meredith insists, but as she pushes up from the recliner, her knees buckle and she falls back. Ginny's arms are around her in an instant. Kathy and Melinda move in to Meredith's other side to help. "We've got you, Mom. It's okay," Kathy assures her. "We'll help you up."

Meredith pulls her arms from her daughters' gentle hold. She sinks back in the chair. Her face contorts and she begins to sob. "I don't want to be a burden!"

Her daughters kneel and wrap their arms around her, assuring her in unison: "You're not a burden, Mom."

Meredith sobs even louder. "Yes, I am. I can't even get up from the chair by myself. I can't make my own meals. I need help to get out of the bed. I even need help to go to the bathroom. I hate this!"

Melinda turns to me. "We try to convince her, but she won't believe she's not a burden."

"You should all be home taking care of your own families," Meredith declares. "Not here, taking care of me."

"We want to be here, Mom."

While they attempt to soothe Meredith, I gaze around the room, at the walls covered with family photos: not the photos from a photographer's studio, but spontaneous photos of grandchildren wild-eyed in an inflatable kiddy pool in Meredith's backyard, of her daughters with arms wrapped around each other at her dining room table, laughing over a lopsided cake blazing with scores of birthday candles. Photo after photo. Happy photos of a happy family.

I turn to Meredith. "I was looking at the photos on your wall."

She looks up.

"I noticed that almost all of them are taken here, at this house."

She studies the photos. "I never noticed that before."

"Your family came here to celebrate," I add, "to be together, even after they were grown."

Meredith's gaze moves along the photos chronicling celebrations and happy times as her daughters grew up, as her grandchildren are growing up. Slowly, she nods.

"I suspect that you were the one making sure everyone had a great time." I point to a photo of her kitchen, where a grinning child stands shrouded in flour, holding aloft a fresh plate of Christmas cookies. "How long did it take you to clean the kitchen after that?"

Her mouth lifts in a wistful smile. "I don't remember . . . but it was worth it."

"You looked after everyone. This is where people came to feel special, to feel loved, to feel happy."

She gazes at the photos, smiling. "I guess so."

"And now, instead of you taking care of the people you love, you need help to take care of yourself."

She bites her lip. Fresh tears spill from her eyes. "I don't want to be a burden," she whispers.

Slowly, I nod.

"It's not fair," she adds, frowning.

"It's hard to accept help."

She nods.

"You raised three daughters. And when they were little, you changed their diapers, cleaned their scraped knees, taught them how to bake, and listened while they sobbed over their first boyfriend. First your daughters, and then your grandchildren. I suspect some of the happiest times of your life are spent taking care of the people you love."

She exhales. "Yes, yes, they are." She turns to her daughters and reaches for their hands. "I'm so proud of each of you. You're good mothers, all of you."

"You taught them that," I say quietly.

Meredith turns to me, her eyes widening.

"They learned that from you. And now you face one of the hardest lessons we all have to learn: that we leave this world much the way we come into it, dependent on others.

"You raised three young women who are all good mothers, who give selflessly, through good times and bad. They, in turn, are teaching this to their children. Someday those children will grow up and have children of their own, who will also learn this love, this caring. This is your legacy, Meredith. As hard as dependence is, it shows us something we might never have seen. It shows us the value of interdependence, that what we do affects others in ways we might never have known. As you go through this time, you can see what you've given in life, because it's returning to you now."

Meredith gazes at her daughters.

"This is their chance to care for you," I offer, "as you have always cared for them. I've watched how they interact with you. They're here not to pay a debt, or because they feel an obligation. For you, it's difficult to accept, but for them, it isn't a burden, it's an act of love."

"It's true," Meredith's daughters declare as they clasp her hands.

"And though dependence is one of the most difficult lessons, I think it's also one of the greatest gifts the end-of-life journey offers.

Through this, perhaps, the true meaning of love can be fully realized. In love, giving and receiving may really be one and the same. When we give with love, we receive love. When we accept and receive something given with love—whether that's support, something tangible, or just kind words—we give love. It's here, Meredith, all around you. It's been a part of you all your life."

Meredith gazes at her daughters, then at the photos that cover the walls. Through tears, she smiles. "This life—" Her voice breaks. "This life . . . all of you have been such a gift."

Human beings, by changing the inner aspects of the mind, can change the outer aspects of their lives.

—William James

The love we give away is the only love we keep.

—Elbert Hubbard

I Wish I Had More Energy . . .

Tools to Maximize Energy and Mobility

Glen and Charlie

"I'M IN NURSING SCHOOL," CHARLIE SAYS as he sits beside his father in the apartment they share. "They let me take a leave so I could be with him. He was pretty mad when I did that. Said I should have stayed in school. But I wouldn't be anywhere else." He turns to his father. "So you're stuck with me, Pops. Just us two bachelors and this nurse who'll come to see us now and then." He grins, trying to coax a smile from his father.

Glen, in his early sixties, manages a brief smile, then lowers his gaze.

Charlie watches his father, his expression hopeful. Earlier I'd learned from the social worker that Charlie is Glen's only child, born when Glen was thirty-nine, a happy and welcome surprise. The marriage didn't last, but his love for his son did. He raised him as a single father and, watching them now, it's clear that their love for each other remains strong.

Charlie turns to me. "Is there something we could do to give Pops a little more energy? He spends most of his time sitting on the couch. I worry about him when I have to go out for groceries or medicine. I'm afraid he'll try to do something he can't, and fall. He can barely walk a few steps without having to grab hold of something. He just doesn't know his limits."

I turn to Glen, watching as he hunches further inward. I suspect that Glen is all too aware of his limits. I turn to Charlie. "What field of nursing do you think you'll choose?"

"Well, I'd been thinking about pediatrics, but spending this time with Pops I realize what a difference I could make in the lives of seniors. They're really underserved. I don't think I could do hospice, though. I don't know how you do it."

I smile. "For me, and for most people who work in hospice, it's an opportunity to help people a lot like your dad regain some of what they've lost because of illness. Of all the things we face in this journey, I think the loss of independence is one of the hardest to deal with. We help people like your dad find ways to regain some of those losses."

From the corner of my eye, I see Glen's head lifting slightly. I continue. "When I visit someone who faces this, I ask him what he enjoys doing that he can no longer do. For example, if he loves to go outside, but can no longer walk long distances, we can bring in a wheelchair. He may still be quite capable of walking, but the wheelchair offers a lot more flexibility and opportunity. It helps him extend his energy and do more. Some people will even use the wheelchair around the house. And though they may still be able to walk, the added safety, combined with the energy they save, is worth the inconvenience of using the wheelchair.

"The most important consideration though, is what the person values. For some, being seen in a wheelchair isn't worth the pleasure of going outside. For some, it's more important to try to make their way around the house, holding on to furniture, hoping they don't fall, rather than using the wheelchair. Bottom line: It's their choice. What's most important to them? What do they value? No one can make that decision for them. Illness can take so much from us. It requires us to make some choices we'd rather not consider. But we *do* have choices."

Gone is the dull expression on Glen's face. His gaze is intent. "So you're saying it's up to me whether I use a wheelchair?"

I nod. "Absolutely."

"Charlie's been telling me I have to use it, that I can't get around anymore without one."

I offer a sympathetic smile. "He's worried about you. He's afraid that, if you fall, you'll really hurt yourself. Right now you can walk, but you have to hold on to furniture to make your way around. I suspect you don't go far. And when you do move around I suspect it wears you out."

Glen's gaze drops. Slowly, he nods. Then he looks up. "Are you saying I could go outside?"

"You can. What else would you like to do?"

He turns to his son. "I'd really like it if you went out sometimes. Just get out of the house. Be with people your own age, not always stuck here with your old man."

"But I like being here with you, Pops."

Glen's lip curls wryly. "You know I love you, but sometimes I just feel smothered with you hovering over me. A little time alone would be nice. I used to be alone all the time, after you graduated from high school and moved out. I love being with you, but I think I'd enjoy it more if I didn't feel the only reason you were staying home was because you thought I needed help, that I couldn't be left alone."

I wait as Charlie takes in Glen's words. Then I ask, "How about this idea, Charlie? If your dad agreed to use a wheelchair while you were out, would you feel he would be safe, that you could leave him and not worry?"

Glen's eyes widen and I add hastily, "Even though you *can* walk, Glen, you would be using it simply to give Charlie peace of mind so he could go out."

I turn back to Charlie. "If your dad agreed to do this, and honored that agreement, do you feel you could go out now and then, and he would be safe?"

Charlie sucks in a breath. "Would you really do that, Pops? Use the wheelchair while I was out?"

Glen considers his question, then nods. "If you would go out and enjoy yourself, then yes, I'd do that for you."

Charlie gazes at his father. Then he smiles. "So you'd let me take you outside, too?"

Glen turns to me, exasperated, and I interject. "I think, Charlie, your dad would enjoy spending time outside with you, using the wheelchair to conserve his energy. But the idea that he's dependent on you isn't much fun."

Charlie's brows furrow. "How's that different from what I said?"

Glen answers. "You know, son, it's hard enough to think about having to use a wheelchair, but if we could go out together and enjoy being out, like we used to, that would be okay. Yes, I'd have to use a wheelchair, and I'd probably need you to push it along, but . . . but the difference is that it's hard for me to think about being dependent on you, that I need you to take me outside." He shrugs. "So when you ask if I'd let you take me outside, I sort of feel like I'm some little kid. Maybe just ask me if I want to go outside." Then Glen shakes his head. "Maybe I'm just kidding myself. Maybe none of this makes sense—"

"Actually, Pops, I think I get what you're saying."

"You do?"

Charlie nods. "If you do decide to use a wheelchair to go out, it's because using it gives you back some of your independence. And it would be more like it used to be, with us just being out together, rather than you needing me to help you."

"I'd really like that."

"You may even choose, Glen, to use the wheelchair around the house, even when Charlie's here. Even though you can get around short distances by holding on to things, it's got to be tiring, and limiting. Using the wheelchair to get around will allow you to go farther and leave you with more energy for the things that matter to you."

Glen considers my words, then nods slowly.

Charlie lays a gentle hand on his dad's knee. "So we could go out for walks again?"

Glen smiles. "I'd like that." Then he adds, "Just not on Tuesdays. Sally, upstairs, has her bridge club on Tuesdays, and I don't want all those lovely ladies to see me in a wheelchair."

Charlie grins. "Any day but Tuesdays."

"I have another idea of something that might help you regain some energy and independence," I add. "Think of energy being like cash in a bank. You have only so much of it. If you have an event coming up that you're looking forward to, like an outing with your son, or Tuesdays, sitting by the window, flirting with all those lovely bridge players as they arrive—"

Charlie grins at his father. "Busted!"

I smile and continue. "You could consider planning for naps. Put a little energy in the bank, so to speak, when you know you have a large withdrawal coming out later. This way you'll be more alert and engaged for the things that matter to you. Again, it's your choice. It's up to you to decide what's worth spending your energy on, what's important to you."

"What do you think, Pops? Do you think that might work for you?"

Glen's brows knit together. Finally, he answers. "A long time ago, long before you were born, I used to play bridge. Maybe I could take a nap Tuesday mornings . . ."

If you lose hope, somehow you lose the vitality that keeps life moving, you lose that courage to be, that quality that helps you go on, in spite of it all. And so today, I still have a dream.

—Martin Luther King, Jr.

Ways to Maximize Your Energy

- Determine what activities you value most.
- For loved ones, recognize that only the affected person can decide what he values most, what he wants to spend his energy on.
- Talk with your health care team about mobility tools, such as four-point canes, walkers, and wheelchairs. A physical therapist can show you how to safely use these tools. See "What Does Hospice Do?" (page 57).
- Explore ways to experience the activities you enjoy through use of mobility tools and energy conservation.
- Arrange the main living area to include a comfortable place, such as a bed or a recliner, to sleep, sit, or visit.
- Ask loved ones to arrange the furniture so you have easy, uncluttered access to commonly used areas. See "How Can I Keep Him Safe?" (page 76).

- Place needed objects—like beverages, snacks, remote controls, reading materials, eyeglasses, tissues, and trash receptacles—within easy reach. Consider buying an extension gripper device to help you reach objects.

- Consider purchasing a one-way monitor or a two-way transmitter (an intercom or a walkie-talkie) to facilitate communication. See "How Can I Keep Him Safe?" (page 76).

- If you will be alone in the home, look into a fall-alert monitoring service, which provides a device, often worn around the neck, that you can press to summon help in the event of a fall.

- Consider adaptive tools, such as a toilet riser and a bath bench. See "How Do I Bring the Bathroom to Him?" (page 85).

- Schedule naps before and after activities.

- Allow for rest days before and after planned active days.

- Encourage visitors to make frequent, short visits, rather than long, infrequent visits. Consider placing a sign on the door that shares your wishes. Fashion the sign in such a way that it can be reversed. One side of the sign might say, "I'm resting now. Please leave a note." Leave a basket beside the door with paper and a pen. The other side of the sign could let people know you're available for a visit, and how much of a visit you're up for. (For example, "Welcome! Please limit your visit to 30 minutes. Thanks.") This sets an expectation and spares you from having to think of a polite way to ask a visitor to leave. If you find that you're able and wish to visit longer, you can ask your visitor to stay.

DO I WANT TO HELP PLAN MY REMEMBRANCE SERVICE?

Ways to Explore This Topic with Loved Ones

Lily

"WHAT DO YOU THINK? TOO MUCH?" Lily asks as she tips her freshly made-up face for inspection.

I smile at the cherry-red lipstick and the bold dash of rouge streaking across her deeply lined face. "Perfect!"

"That's what I thought." She casts a rueful glance at the gray clouds and drizzle outside her window. "On a day like today, a lady needs all the color she can get."

"Hi, Mom," a chorus of Lily's children call out as they enter the room, each bending for a hug and a kiss, each wiping the bright smear of lipstick from their cheek as they settle on a corner of Lily's queen-sized bed. Her children are, in fact, older adults, each with adult children of their own.

"Well," Lily announces, "I've asked you all to come today because I have something important I want to do. I want to plan a party for after I'm gone. Call it a celebration of life, call it a cheerful funeral, call it a remembrance service, whatever you like, but I've been happy nearly every day of my life, and I'd like to be remembered that way, too."

Her children's eyes widen. "Well, Mom," says Tom, her eldest. "We can do that now, but are you sure you want to?"

"Absolutely! Why wouldn't I?"

"Well, it's kind of a depressing topic," offers her daughter Daisy. "And besides, I'd rather enjoy you now. I don't want to think about that time after you're gone."

Lily shakes her head. "But I *will* be gone. Maybe soon. And I don't want to leave this for you, to try to do immediately after I go. This way we're not in a big hurry. We can take a little time to plan what we want, and shop around. And besides, by planning now, I get to have a say in what I want."

Slowly, Lily's children nod, but their faces reveal their apprehension. Ignoring this, Lily continues. "When I was young, when someone died you had a funeral. It was dark, and solemn, and people cried. I don't want that. To me, the best part of every day was to make someone happy, to make each of you happy. And yes, when someone we love dies, we're sad. But I think we're sad because that person brought something special to our lives, brought out something good in us, and we'll miss them. But what I want is for you, for my friends, to remember the happiness we shared, the love we shared. That kind of event may not be right for everyone, but it's right for me. That's just who I am."

"That's true enough," says Rose, the youngest. "You always—" Her voice breaks. "You always saw the bright side of things."

"Shhhh . . ." Lily reaches to Rose and wipes a tear away. "No tears. I'm glad to have lived this life. I will miss you, but this is life. It ends. And yes, you will be sad, and I know you'll cry, but I want you to come together that day, not to cry, but to remember how happy we've all been together. And I want you to go forward, after I'm gone, and live with that happiness still a part of you. And that way," she squeezes Rose's hand, "I'll still be with you. The best part of me will still be here."

"But Mom—"

"No," she wags her finger at Tom. "No arguments. What made me happiest was to help the people around me be happy, too. That's what I want for that day. Will you help me make that happen?"

A long silence follows. Then, one by one, her children come forward for a long, tight hug. "Of course we will."

Together they choose music that reflects Lily's bright spirit. They also choose passages from their scripture that best represent Lily's view of life. Rose suggests that each of the siblings write something to share that day, their favorite memories that show what their mom taught them about life, about laughter, about love. "If we have to stand and read it, we can't cry," she reasons, laughing.

Lily shares that she'd like her body cremated, with her ashes scattered in her garden. "That way I'll be a part of something growing, something that continues to give joy, to nurture long after I'm gone." Her children visibly stiffen. She smiles. "It's what happens. My spirit will fly, but the body remains, and you have to do something with it."

Slowly, Tom nods. "Okay." Then he smiles. "You know, I'm really glad you told us this. I wouldn't have known what to do, what you would have wanted, and this way . . . This way we know it's what you want."

Lily smiles. "Exactly!" Then she asks, "Who wants to read my letter that day?"

Her children's eyes widen.

"You didn't really think I wouldn't have something to say, did you?"

"No, that would be a first," Tom laughs. "Even when I didn't like what you had to say, I knew—most of the time anyway—that you were right." He sighs. "You've always had this clear, uncluttered way of seeing a situation."

Lily shrugs. "I guess I've always believed, when you get right down to it, that life is pretty simple. Just be kind. You can't change what other people do, but if you're kind, the rest doesn't matter. And maybe that's all I'll say in my letter. Be kind."

She reaches for her children's hands. "Be kind. Be happy."

What you leave behind is not what is engraved in stone monuments, but what is woven into the lives of others.

Pericles

IDEAS FOR PLANNING A REMEMBRANCE SERVICE

A remembrance service incorporates an acknowledgment of the death, an opportunity for remembrance, and may also include a disposition of the remains, through burial of the body, or a scattering or interring of the ashes. If you opt for cremation, your ashes can also be scattered at a later date, at a location chosen by you or your loved ones.

If you decide to participate in planning your service, choose who you want to assist you in planning. You may wish to include loved ones, as this service is for them as well. If you've been active in a religious organization, consider involving your spiritual leader, too.

What structure do you want for the event? For example:

+ Do you want a traditional service, incorporating traditions of your faith?
+ Do you want a nontraditional service? If so, describe what that means to you.
+ What theme or message do you want to convey to reflect your views on the meaning of your life?

What elements do you want to incorporate to express that theme? Ideas might include:

+ Readings from scripture or a poem
+ A self-composed letter to be read on your behalf
+ Readings composed by loved ones, sharing memories of your time together
+ Musical selections

Where would you like the service or gathering held? Ideas might include:

+ A place of worship
+ An outdoor location, such as a garden, a clearing in the woods, or beside a body of water, such as a lake, river, or ocean
+ A community center or your home

Do you want to ask your friends and loved ones to honor your memory by making a donation to your favorite charity, or a charity of their choice?

Do you have a favorite photo of yourself you'd like published in a formal program?

Do you want to include a message in the program to reflect your personality and values? Ideas might include:

+ A poem
+ A passage of scripture
+ A favorite quote
+ A drawing or photo

Do you have a preference for either cremation or burial of your body?

Where would you like your remains to rest? Consider talking with loved ones about this, as some loved ones might want to be able to visit the location where your remains rest. If you choose cremation and want your ashes to be scattered, ask a funeral home representative about applicable laws governing the scattering of human ashes.

Have you made prior financial arrangements for burial or cremation? If so, put the documents with your other important papers. See "Appendix B: Important Documents to Gather" (page 215).

Consider shopping for funeral services in advance. Prices vary widely for identical services and products. Keep in mind that cremation is often significantly less expensive than burial of a body.

Finally, communicate your wishes verbally and in writing. A written description will help your loved ones avoid confusion or conflict at the time of passing.

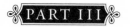

❧ PART III ❧

Caregiving as a Family:
How Do We Manage?

This section offers information that may be helpful for loved ones and caregivers. Individuals coping with declining health may find value in some of this material, as well.

In this section you'll learn how to adapt to physical decline. You'll find suggestions to maximize mobility, energy, and safety; advice for adapting to a changing appetite; tips for gathering and organizing help; and information about available resources, including hospice. You'll learn about how to manage communication and minimize conflict within your family. You'll also find guidance for selecting a care facility, if caregiving at home is no longer possible. Each chapter is followed by extensive checklists and other tools for quick and easy reference.

I've Never Done This Before . . .
An Overview of Caregiving

What Does Hospice Do?
An Explanation of Services
Why Early Access to Hospice Can Help You and Your Loved Ones

What If We Don't Have Hospice Care?
Tips for Accessing Resources
Making the Most of Your Visit with Your Doctor
Guidance for Managing Care in a Rural Community

I Can't Do This Alone . . .
Suggestions to Gather, Organize, and Manage Support from Friends,
Neighbors, and Loved Ones

How Can I Keep Him Safe?
Understanding and Reducing Risks for Both the Individual and the Caregiver

How Do I Bring the Bathroom to Him?
Options for Toileting and Bathing

I Don't Know What to Say . . .
Insights to Achieve a Meaningful Visit

He Doesn't Want to Eat . . .
Understanding and Adapting to a Changing Appetite
Ideas for Adapting Meal Schedules for People with Memory Impairment
Suggestions for Easy-to-Digest Foods and Beverages

For Loved Ones Who Live Far Away: What Can I Do?
Staying Informed and Supportive
Deciding When to Visit

I'm Exhausted! Exploring Care Settings Outside the Home
Choosing a Care Facility, If Needed, and Paying for Care

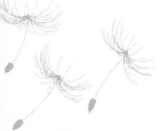

❀ I've Never Done This Before . . . ❀
An Overview of Caregiving

Clayton and Patty

"I HAVE NO IDEA WHAT TO DO," PATTY CONFIDES. "We knew someday one of us might have to take care of the other, but truthfully, we just avoided talking about it. And now . . ." She reaches across the kitchen table and takes hold of my hand. "I've never taken care of anyone like this before. I have no idea what to expect, what to do . . ." In the next room Clayton, her husband, new to hospice with a life expectancy of about six months, sleeps in his recliner.

Gently, I squeeze her fingers. "I suspect you're both pretty scared."

Tears well up in her eyes. "I just don't know if I can do this . . . I want to, I want him to stay home, I want to take care of him, but . . . I think not knowing what to expect is the hardest. If I had some idea of what we were facing, I think I'd be able to deal with it better."

"If you think it will be helpful, I can offer you a general idea of some of the issues families face as they care for a loved one at home."

"That would be helpful. Just to know what lies ahead will make this a lot less frightening."

"So let's take a look at that. But if you and Clayton decide that being at home becomes too difficult, there are good alternatives, and we can help locate a place where he can be cared for, where you're both comfortable."

EVERYONE IS UNIQUE

Remember, everyone is unique, and every family does this their own way, based on their values and situation. Also be aware that, over time, things will change and you'll need to adapt the care—of both him and you—with those changes. With each change we'll talk in greater detail as the need arises. For now, let's just look at the big picture.

Managing with Declining Mobility

One of the biggest issues you'll both face is his declining mobility. Right now he gets around pretty well. Over time, he'll likely become weaker, and may be at risk of falling. You can adapt things in the home and bring in equipment—maybe a four-point cane, or a walker or wheelchair—to help with that. The real issue, however, is that Clayton is an independent man. It won't be easy for him to ask for things, or to ask you to help him get up and move around. And frankly, it won't be easy for you to help him. He's bigger than you are. We need to keep you safe, too. When that time comes, when he needs help getting around, we'll go into a lot more detail about adaptations and safety for both him and you.

Adapting the Bathroom

With declining mobility come some other challenges, like using the bathroom. You can adapt the bathroom with things like a bench for the shower, and what's called a toilet riser. It fits over the toilet. It has handrails and raises the level of the seat to make it easier to sit down and get up again. You can find these things in a medical supply store or buy them used. You might also consider installing safety bars in the bathroom, especially if these bars will help you as well.

Later he may not be able to get to the bathroom, to shower or toilet. If that happens, you'll need to bring the bathroom to him, using a urinal or a bedside commode. The bedside commode is a sturdy chair with handholds and a removable basin. Think of it as a portable toilet.

As for bathing, if it's no longer safe for him to use the shower bench, you'll need to bring the bath to him. A nurse's aide can come to your home and give him a bath or, if you prefer, you can do it. We'll talk about these things in more detail later, if he needs them. For now, just know that if he's no longer able to get around in the bathroom, we can help you adapt to keep both him and you safe.

Maximizing His Energy

Over time it's likely that he'll begin to sleep more. At first, he might be happiest just napping in your bedroom. Later, when he has less energy, and may even need help getting around, you might consider setting up a bed in the living area, where you spend the most time, either turning the couch into a bed or bringing in a hospital bed. A bed in the living area gives him a comfortable place, near everyone, where he can join in conversations, or just rest. You'll probably be more comfortable there, too. You can talk to him while you're nearby, and have a comfortable place to sit with him throughout the day.

Adapting to a Changing Appetite

It's likely he'll experience a decrease in appetite and a change in food preferences. If he does, we'll want to explore why. Though a diminished appetite is a normal part of the process, sometimes it's caused by things we can treat, like difficulty or discomfort swallowing, which may be brought on by an infection. It may also be caused by fatigue. Some people with heart or lung problems can get really short of breath while eating. If that's the case, a change to soft foods can help minimize this challenge.

Other treatable causes of decreased appetite include nausea and constipation. For nausea, we can try different foods, or medication. For constipation, the best strategy is to prevent it. Because of the medicine he takes and his decreased activity, he's at high risk for constipation. You'll want to keep track of bowel movements, maybe keep a pen and a calendar or notebook in the bathroom. If more than two days pass without a bowel movement, you'll need to increase the amount of laxatives he takes. If this happens, call hospice and we can offer guidance.

There are medicines that can, at least temporarily, stimulate appetite. They work well, up to a point. Later in the process, when someone has perhaps only a few weeks, these medicines aren't effective and might even be counterproductive.

Another way to address decreasing appetite is to offer smaller meals and frequent snacks. His food preferences might also change. He may not want to eat much meat, but may enjoy more easily digested foods, like soups, mashed potatoes, custards, nutritional drinks—things like that.

At the same time, *you* need to eat. And you won't have a lot of time to spend cooking, so we need to develop a plan where you can keep things on hand for both you and him.

Understanding and Preventing Delirium

You should probably know about delirium, even though it may never be an issue. Delirium has a number of causes, many of which are preventable or easily resolved, so knowing how to prevent it, or how to recognize the early signs, can be helpful.

Basically, delirium is a sudden onset of confusion. Someone may be thinking quite clearly, and within hours he may become unable to focus, have a conversation, or follow basic instructions. Delirium is different from dementia, which is confusion caused by gradual memory loss, with changes occurring over months or years. With delirium, you'll notice changes in his ability to think and interact within a matter of hours or overnight.

In some cases, people experiencing delirium can become quite active, agitated, or even combative. These cases are fairly easy to recognize. A little more difficult to spot are the cases when the person experiencing delirium becomes quiet or withdrawn. In either case, if you notice a sudden change in mental status or behavior, call hospice.

Delirium can be caused by a variety of problems, including constipation, urinary retention, dehydration, lack of sleep, low oxygen levels, low blood sugar, infection, head trauma from a fall, electrolyte imbalances, adverse reactions to medications, or sudden withdrawal from smoking, alcohol, or a medication. It can be caused by significant changes in routine or environment. It can also be caused by decreases in sensory input, such as not being able to see or hear well for long periods. In all these situations, the goal is to prevent the onset of delirium, or to recognize it early and treat the cause, if possible.

Delirium can also be caused by the disease process. In these cases, the goal would be to treat the symptoms, rather than the cause.

But back to what you can do in the home to prevent it: Basically, you'll want to prevent constipation, offer adequate fluids, and make sure that the home environment is adapted for his needs. This may include keeping a calendar and clock within visual range, maintaining soft lighting, ensuring that he uses his glasses or hearing aides, and maintaining a calm environment with minimal changes in routine. It also helps to keep the mind actively engaged. Rather than watching TV all the time, it's a good idea for him to engage in conversations several times a day.

If he falls, call us immediately. If he has trouble sleeping or is sleeping all day and restless at night, has pain or difficulty when urinating, fever, or any other problems, let us know. And if you do see sudden changes in behavior, call us.

Caregiving as Needs Increase

When he's close to passing, it's likely he'll need total care. He probably won't be able to use a urinal or the bedside commode, so he'll need disposable underwear.

It's also likely that he won't have the strength to turn or reposition himself in bed without help. He'll need help turning about every two hours, around the clock, so he's not uncomfortable, or at risk of developing a pressure wound.

Finding and Managing Help with Caregiving

Caregiving is a big job, and it will be very difficult for you to do alone. You'll need to take care of yourself, too. It's important for you to have quality time with him, for you to be a wife, and not just a caregiver. For that reason, it's important to accept help from your friends, family, and the community.

As word gets out, your friends and neighbors are going to offer to help. I'll point you to some resources and give you a few tips on how to organize that help. But most importantly, you need to become comfortable accepting their offers of help. A lot of people find themselves caring for a loved one. Many don't want to ask for help. But imagine if this were happening to your neighbor or a friend. What would you do? What would you *want* to do?

People really *do* want to help. We live in a culture of independence, but the truth is, that spirit of generosity, of compassion, of just plain neighborliness, still exists. It's there in the people who ask, "How can I help?"

Being independent, it may not be easy to accept this help. But as you're beginning to see, caring for a loved one at home is a demanding job. It's incredibly rewarding, but it's also challenging and tiring. You'll find it will be much easier for both of you if you can accept the help people want to give.

When we reach the end of life, things often become pretty clear. It's the simple things that matter most. This is the time when we realize just how much having good friends and good relationships with our children, giving of ourselves, and being a part of a community matter. These things matter not because of what others can do for us in our time of need, but because of the happiness we've found by sharing love and kindness with others. And now, others are here to share and give with that same feeling of love and kindness.

The future comes one day at a time.

—Dean Acheson

ADDITIONAL CAREGIVING INFORMATION

Parts III and V of this guide offer additional, in-depth caregiving information.

For more specific information about:

Maximizing energy, see "I Wish I Had More Energy . . ." (page 37).

Maximizing safety for the individual and caregivers, see "How Can I Keep Him Safe?" (page 76).

Managing bathing and toileting, see "How Do I Bring the Bathroom to Him?" (page 85).

Adapting to a changing appetite, see "He Doesn't Want to Eat . . ." (page 96).

Addressing emotional and spiritual issues, see Part IV, "Closure: Will I Die a "Good" Death? (page 123).

Caregiving support, see "I Can't Do This Alone . . ." (page 71).

Caregiving in the final days, see "How Do We Keep Her Comfortable?" (page 158).

Hiring caregiving help, see "I'm Exhausted! Exploring Care Settings Outside the Home . . ." (page 112).

Hospice resources, see "What Does Hospice Do?" (page 57).

❧ What Does Hospice Do? ❧

An Explanation of Services
Why Early Access to Hospice Can Help You
and Your Loved Ones

Sid and Marge

SID GLANCES AT HIS WIFE, MARGE, AND squeezes her hand as they sit close together in their living room. At their feet, their dog Barney, an old Labrador, sleeps.

"What does it mean if . . . if I choose hospice?" Sid asks in a shaky voice. "What does hospice do?"

"I'm here to explain what hospice does, and what it can do for you. But it's up to you to decide if it's the right choice for you and your family."

Slowly, Sid nods.

"What's your understanding of your illness?" I ask.

Tears well up in Marge's eyes. Sid's gaze drops. Finally, he answers. "My doctor says my heart just isn't keeping up, even with all the medicines. We've tried them all, and nothing is really helping anymore." He takes a deep breath. "He said . . . He said that I probably only had a few more months before my heart just gave out."

I wait, then ask: "Your doctor shared this with you, but do you feel that's the situation?"

He closes his eyes and draws in several slow, deep breaths. Finally, he opens his eyes. "Yes, we've done all we can to try to get this heart to work the way it should. Maybe I could get a new heart, but—" He shakes his head. "I'm not up to that. I don't want to go through that. All that pain . . . Being in the hospital again . . ." He looks at Marge. "I'd rather be here, with you, in our home." He swallows back the tears that begin to flow. Then he turns to me. "I don't want to die hooked up to machines in a hospital, surrounded by strangers."

Slowly, I nod. Then I turn to Marge. "What about you? How do you feel about this?"

Marge attempts a smile. "I want what Sid wants."

Sid laughs and Barney raises his head at the sound. "You heard her," Sid jokes. "That's got to be the first time in sixty-two years she's said that!" He smiles at Marge. "And I have a witness, too."

Marge nuzzles Sid's shoulder. "You know what I mean."

He offers a tender smile. "I know, sweetheart, but I still love to hear you laugh." Then he turns to me. "So if we choose hospice, what can you do for us?"

"It sounds like your goal is to pursue treatment for comfort, for quality of life, but not for a cure. Is that right?"

Sid nods. "Yes, that's exactly what I want, but I have a lot of questions . . ."

How Can Hospice Help?

Hospice can help you figure out ways to maximize your quality of life, to manage your care here at home, or someplace else, if that's what you decide. We work with your doctor to manage the medicines to keep you comfortable and give you as much energy as possible. We help you and your loved ones adapt, to maximize you abilities, to pursue what's important to you throughout this process.

Through it all, you're in charge. You tell us what your goals are, how you would like this stage of life to play out, and we do our best to help make them happen.

What Can I Hope For?

That's up to you. You tell us what *quality of life* means to you. Each person has their own vision of what that means, and, over time, that vision changes. We can help you explore what holds meaning for you and your loved ones, and help you to enrich the time that remains and live each day to the fullest.

Does My Insurance Pay for Hospice?

Hospice is paid for by the Medicare Part A benefit. Many private insurance companies also pay for hospice care.

What Does Hospice Provide?

Your doctor remains in charge of your care, and we'll work with him to maximize your comfort and quality of life.

Hospice provides a team that comes to you. We bring nurses, social workers, nurse's aides, volunteers, and, if you like, chaplains, too. We all work together to listen and support you and your family.

If you do choose hospice, a nurse will visit you regularly. We'll check you out physically, listen to your concerns, provide emotional support, and keep in touch with your doctor. In addition to visiting you regularly, we're also available twenty-four hours a day, every day of the year for emergencies and questions that can't wait until regular office hours.

Hospice pays for the medications related to your primary diagnosis, and any other medications you need to keep you comfortable. By primary diagnosis, we mean the disease that's causing your decline. In your case, your primary diagnosis is heart disease.

Unfortunately, hospice doesn't pay for medicines unrelated to the primary diagnosis. For example, we don't pay for your thyroid medicine because it's not for your heart, or to help keep you comfortable. But we may be able to find additional resources to help with expenses like that.

In addition to a nurse, you'll also be supported by a social worker. For many families, the costs of a long illness can put a real strain on finances. The social worker can help look into resources you may be eligible for to help pay for other medications, supplement drinks, or other things you might need that hospice doesn't provide.

Hospice also pays for any equipment you might need, like a wheelchair, a walker, or a hospital bed. If you need a physical therapist to help you learn how to use the walker, or any other adaptive devices, hospice will arrange and pay for that, too. Hospice also pays for medical supplies—things like dressings or catheters—if you need them.

Hospice can also provide nurse's aides to visit periodically, to help with baths and other personal care. For some people, one of the hardest things to cope with is the loss of independence. We know you don't have as much energy as you'd like, and no one but you can decide how to spend that energy. Having someone help with your bath will conserve energy that you can then spend on other things. It's your choice.

We also have volunteers available for four hours a week to help out, or just to visit. There may come a time when you need someone to be here all the time. Being alone when you don't have much energy, and it's not longer safe for you to get around without help, can be frightening. A volunteer can give your family a chance to leave the house without leaving you alone.

Hospice also offers a longer rest period called a *respite benefit*. Let's say Marge needs some rest for longer than four hours. Hospice can arrange for someone to come to your home, or for you to get good care somewhere else, like a care facility, for up to five days at a time. Caregiving can be challenging, and we're here to support your family, too.

This time is also emotionally challenging. Hospice isn't just about keeping you physically comfortable. We also provide emotional and, if you choose, spiritual support for you and your family. You'll be supported by a social worker who is trained in counseling. You can also choose to have a chaplain visit. It's up to you. Chaplains provide nondenominational support. Their training encompasses all the major spiritual practices, as well as those common to the area. Like all of us, chaplains will listen and help you explore your own spiritual beliefs, without interjecting their own views. We're all here to help support *your* goals, not our own.

Keep in mind that even if you don't want all that help now, you can always change your mind, at any time, about any of this. Situations change. We're continuously adapting to meet changing needs and wishes.

Do I Really Need Hospice Now?

A lot of people wait, sometimes until the last few weeks or days. Then, when things get really difficult, they call in hospice. When we come in earlier in the process, we have the chance to help families in many ways, physically *and* emotionally. To enable someone to be more comfortable, or to eat what she wants, or sleep better, or have more energy, can make a big difference in her quality of life. When people feel better, they're better able to cope with other important issues, like addressing unfinished business, attaining closure, and rediscovering hope for things that matter most to them.

We can help families find comfort and peace. But if they wait until the last few weeks or days to start this help, it's really difficult, if not impossible, to do all that. The earlier we can help a family, the more significantly we can improve everyone's quality of life.

I Always Thought Choosing Hospice Meant "Giving Up." Is It?

For some people, hospice isn't the right choice. But for others, there are no more treatments, no more surgeries, no more medicines that might offer a cure. For still others, the consequences of pursuing additional treatment or surgery may just be more than they want to go through. For them, and as you've said, for you, the focus turns to comfort, to living the best you can, for whatever time remains. If you want to be able to go outside and enjoy the sunshine, hospice helps figure out how. If you want to have enough energy to enjoy a visit with your grandchildren, hospice helps figure that out. If you want to sit with someone and talk about your hopes and fears, hospice does that, too. Hospice is about helping you and your loved ones cope with the challenges and enjoy the best possible quality of life.

The world is round, and the place which may seem like the end may also be the beginning.

—Ivy Baker Priest

FREQUENTLY ASKED QUESTIONS

How do I get hospice care?

You must be referred to hospice by a doctor. Talk with your doctor about your wishes. If you meet the medical guidelines, your doctor will make the referral to hospice.

Where is hospice provided?

Hospice is most commonly provided in the home, but can also be provided in a long-term-care facility, a group residence, or an adult foster home. Hospice can also be provided on a short-term basis in a hospital or an inpatient specialty hospice, based on medical need.

What are the medical guidelines for hospice eligibility?

You may be eligible for hospice care if your doctor feels that if your disease runs its normal, expected course, you have a life expectancy of about six months, and if you choose the care of hospice rather than other treatments for this illness.

I'd like the extra support that hospice provides, but my doctor says I don't meet the medical guidelines. What can I do?

Some communities offer support similar to hospice, called palliative care. Palliative care, like hospice, focuses on relief of pain and other symptoms of serious illness. The goal is to prevent or ease suffering, and to offer individuals and their families the best possible quality of life. Unlike hospice, palliative care is appropriate at any stage of a serious illness and is not dependent on life expectancy. It can be provided at the same time as curative or life-prolonging treatment. For more information about palliative care, see "Appendix A: Additional Resources" (page 210).

You may also qualify for home health support. Talk with your health care provider about available options.

I think hospice might be right for me, but my doctor seems resistant. What can I do to get her to consider hospice?

Make an appointment with your doctor. Let the office staff know you want time to discuss your treatment options. Be prepared to discuss why you want to discontinue curative treatment and change to comfort-focused care.

At the visit, share your wishes with your doctor. If the doctor is still resistant, ask for an explanation and continue the discussion until you feel satisfied with the outcome.

Who pays for hospice?

In the United States, hospice care is paid for through the Medicare Part A benefit. Medicaid and many other health insurance providers pay for hospice care as well. Talk with your policy representative to learn more. In many other countries, hospice care is part of the national health plan.

Can I get hospice care if I don't have health insurance?

Yes. You may be asked to pay privately for the care. If you have limited funds, you may qualify for financial assistance. To qualify for this assistance, you may be required to complete an application demonstrating your financial need.

If I sign up for hospice, can I change my mind?

Yes. Medicare recipients can choose to end hospice care and pursue other treatments. If, at a later date, they choose to start hospice again, they can. This will vary for other insurance policies.

What do hospice nurses do?

Hospice nurses regularly visit individuals in their home or other care setting. We assess the person's physical status and update the physician, requesting medication changes, as needed. We teach caregivers about medications and caregiving issues. We assess for potential problems, and provide instruction about what to do should the problem arise. We are available by phone at all times for emergencies.

We also listen to concerns, including emotional or spiritual issues, and work with the individual and others on the hospice team to help resolve these issues. Our goal is to support individuals and families, without interjecting our beliefs or values.

What does a Medicare-certified hospice provide?

- Doctors' services for the terminal illness
- Nurses' services
- Social work services
- Chaplain services
- Nurse's aide and housekeeping services
- Volunteer services
- Physical, occupational, and speech therapy
- Dietary counseling
- Medical equipment
- Medical supplies
- Medications for symptom control or pain relief (may require a small co-payment)
- Hospitalization for symptom relief if preapproved by your hospice
- Short-term respite care
- Grief and loss support

What doesn't a Medicare-certified hospice pay for?

- Curative treatment
- Medications not for comfort or symptom relief
- Treatment not arranged by the hospice
- Room and board
- Personal items, such as tissues, disposable underwear, etc.
- Nutritional supplements, unless prescribed by your doctor
- Emergency room visits, unless preapproved by the hospice
- Ambulance transportation, unless arranged by the hospice

What does hospice provide in the United Kingdom?
 ◆ Basic medical and nursing care, including rehabilitation,
   physiotherapies, and complementary therapies to achieve pain and
   symptom control
 ◆ Spiritual support
 ◆ Practical and financial advice
 ◆ Bereavement support
This care can be provided in the home, in a hospice facility, or in a
hospital.

For more information about hospice care in the UK, see "Appendix A:
Additional Resources" (page 210).

What does hospice provide in Canada?
 ◆ Basic medical care
 ◆ Medications for symptom control, pain relief, or improved quality of
   life, provided they are on the program formulary
 ◆ Medical equipment and supplies necessary to provide safe and high-
   quality palliative care
 ◆ Counseling and social support
 ◆ Respite care
 ◆ Volunteer support
For more information about hospice care in Canada, see "Appendix A:
Additional Resources" (page 210).

To locate hospice services in other countries, see "Appendix A: Additional
Resources" (page 210).

What if We Don't Have Hospice Care?

Tips for Accessing Resources
Making the Most of Your Visit with Your Doctor
Guidance for Managing Care in a Rural Community

Marianne and Greg

"I'm not sure it's a good idea," Greg shares. "We won't have access to hospice care, but it's what she wants. She was raised there, and it's where she's happiest. She wants to spend her last months looking out on pastures, not concrete. I can't blame her."

Greg has taken a leave from his job and will move his wife, Marianne, and their young family back to Marianne's parents' farm. A dedicated rural doctor has agreed to care for Marianne and support the family through this process.

"Let's consider what resources are available, and some of the challenges you might face," I offer. "Then let's develop a plan to access those resources and prevent as many problems as possible."

"Boy, that would be helpful. Truthfully, I'm a little scared about this. It's a lot to take on. But I want to do this for her. I just . . . I'm just afraid of being out there, on my own. Can we really do this? Without hospice? In a rural community?"

Gathering Resources

It will be helpful to have Internet access in your home. You won't have a lot of time to sit at the computer, but Internet access can help you locate organizations and agencies that can provide some support. Using the Internet, you can research what they offer.

You'll also want to develop a network of people within the community who can help. Churches, civic organizations, and community centers are all good places to get the word out that you'd welcome help. Make a list of things you'd like help with, and share that list when people offer their help.

One of the challenges you'll face in a rural community is the distance and time involved in getting prescriptions, groceries, and medical supplies. Ask your neighbors if they'd be willing to pick things up for you. People in rural communities often have a regular schedule for going into town. Mark these days on a calendar, along with the person's phone number, so you can call the day before with a list of what you need. Or ask your neighbors to call you before trips, to see if you need anything.

You'll want to keep a week or more of supplies and medicines on hand. In most cases you can anticipate your needs, but for new prescriptions that you need right away, when you can't wait for mail order, you can arrange for someone you know who's going into town to pick up the medicine. It's a good idea to call the pharmacy ahead of time. Make sure they have the medication on hand, and if so, tell them who will be picking it up for you.

Arranging for Medical Equipment

Another issue you'll need to deal with is medical equipment. Many regional offices of national support agencies, like the American Cancer Society, lend medical equipment. Contact the nearest office and inquire about equipment and other support they may have available. In many cases you'll need to pick up and return the equipment, but you can ask a friend to do that on his next trip into the city. Another good source for locating medical equipment is craigslist, a free, Internet classified service. Here you might find used medical equipment for sale nearby, at a reasonable price.

Working with Your Pharmacist

Given that you won't have a hospice nurse coming to visit and answer questions, you'll want to develop good sources of information. Pharmacists are great resources. They can answer questions and address concerns about medications, dosages, side effects—things like that. Compile a list of Marianne's medications, along with dosages, and ask the pharmacist to look it over. Your pharmacist can also be very helpful in problem solving with the doctor when new symptoms occur, or if a medication isn't working as well as you'd like.

Talk with the pharmacist about options for getting medications in an after-hours emergency. If you do have an emergency, having a pharmacist who's familiar with the situation will help a lot.

Working with Your Doctor

Rural doctors are used to the challenges of caring for people who live in the country. They're usually very good at anticipating what medications will be needed, and prescribing them to have on hand, so you're not trying to get them in an emergency, when the pharmacy is closed.

And while most rural doctors aren't specialists, they're generally quite resourceful when it comes to gathering information. In addition to other sources, the doctor can contact the city hospital's Palliative Care Department, or he can contact a hospice medical director. Most hospice medical directors and palliative care specialists are more than happy to share their knowledge.

Also, you'll want to make the most of your visits with the doctor. Keep a list of questions and issues you want to talk about, and bring it to each visit. You'll also want to bring the list of Marianne's medications, and a log of how much and when she takes each one. Show the doctor these lists. If her pain changes in any way, talk with him about that, too.

You'll want to bring along the record of her bowel movements. If the doctor adjusts the pain medication, the dose of the laxatives will need to be adjusted, too. Being able to look at the record and see how the current dosages are working will help the doctor fine-tune the amount.

It's a good idea to take notes at the visit, or bring someone with you to listen and take notes. There's a lot to take in, and sometimes you might not catch it all. Having someone else there can be very helpful.

Also, be sure to raise any concerns you have. Ask "what if" questions.

These are especially important when you have limited support. If an adverse situation is likely to occur, you need to know what to do, and have the tools and medicines on hand to deal with the problem, should it arise.

And, finally, repeat the instructions the doctor gives you, to be sure you understand them correctly.

LEARNING NEW SKILLS

You'll need to learn some new skills—caregiving skills. You might want to do some reading on the subject. You can also ask around in the community. I suspect that many of your neighbors have gone through something like this before and will be happy to share their knowledge with you.

And remember, as difficult as this might be, it's also an opportunity to spend some wonderful, meaningful time together in a peaceful place that holds meaning for you both.

One doesn't discover new lands without consenting to lose sight of the shore for a very long time.

—André Gide

GATHERING SUPPORT WHEN HOSPICE SERVICES ARE NOT AVAILABLE

- Develop a network of volunteer support within your community. For more information, see "I Can't Do This Alone . . ." (page 71).
- Utilize the Internet to research organizations that might offer resources or assistance. For more information, see "Appendix A: Additional Resources" (page 210).
- Talk with your insurance representative about the benefits available to you through your health insurance plan.
- In rural settings, have at least a week or more of supplies and medications on hand at all times.
- Provide relevant information to local health care professionals who will be involved in providing care, including your local pharmacist.

- Make the most of your visits with your doctor:

  Write down questions and concerns as they occur, and bring this list with you to your visit.

  Keep a detailed record of your medication use. See "Will I Be in Pain?" (page 26) for more information. Share this record with your doctor.

  Keep a record of bowel movements and laxative use. Share this with your doctor.

  Take notes, or bring someone with you to listen and take notes.

  Ask questions. Work with your doctor to anticipate problems and have a plan for addressing them.

  Repeat the instructions your doctor gives you to make sure you understand these instructions correctly.

  With your doctor and pharmacist, develop a plan for obtaining medications in an after-hours emergency.

- Read Parts III ("Caregiving as a Family: How Do We Manage?") and V ("For Loved Ones and Caregivers: Sharing the Final Days") of this guide for additional information about caregiving. Ask neighbors experienced in caregiving to offer instruction.

- To locate additional caregiving resources, see "Appendix A: Additional Resources" (page 210).

❀ I Can't Do This Alone ... ❀

Suggestions to Gather, Organize, and Manage Support from Friends, Neighbors, and Loved Ones

Mel and Abby

"I'M JUST SO TIRED . . . I'M GLAD HE'S HERE, in our home, but I'm not sure how much longer I can keep doing this." Abby sighs. "Do you have any magic tricks that can help us?"

I offer a gentle smile. "You could call it magic. I think it's one of the most wonderful things we can experience at a time like this. As time goes by and the person's needs increase, caregiving can become an overwhelming job, but there are ways to deal with it—ways that can improve not only your lives, but the lives of others as well.

"I suspect a lot of your neighbors have asked what they can do to help, or have asked you to let them know if you need help."

"They have."

"What do you tell them?"

"I don't want to burden them. They have their own lives, their own things to deal with."

I nod, then ask, "What would you do if your positions were reversed, if your neighbor told you her husband was seriously ill?"

Abby's eyes widen. Then she smiles. "I'd want to help, but it's a lot easier to give help than it is to ask for it."

"It's that way for many people. But the truth is that the people who offer really do want to help. I spend a lot of time around people at this time in their lives. Quite often they'll share what has made them happiest. Some people will list things—possessions or professional accomplishments. They'll say 'I did this' or 'I have that . . .' But there are many who share that what has made them happiest is helping someone else live a better life, or realize their potential. Generosity, kindness, compassion, doing something to help others can provide a real sense of purpose or meaning.

"Yes, it's difficult to ask for help," I add, "But by asking, by accepting help, you give them something as well. You give them a chance to make a real difference."

"You're saying I should ask my friends, neighbors, and the church members for help?"

"I'm saying that a few moments ago you said you didn't know how much longer you could do this alone. I'm saying that if you offer your friends and neighbors a chance to help, you're giving them a chance to enrich their lives, too. In accepting help, you may be better able to care for Mel at home. You'll also be better able to be a wife and not just an exhausted caregiver."

Abby considers my words. Then, slowly, she nods. "How do I ask? And, frankly, what do I ask for?"

How to Ask for Help

Choose a few friends and a neighbor or two, and let them know that things are becoming a little overwhelming. Let them know that if anyone wanted to help, you'd welcome the support. You also mentioned your church. Let them know, too. Word will get out. People will ask what they can do.

What Would Be Helpful to You?

Let's put together a list of tasks you need help with. For a lot of people going through this, cooking is a real chore. They don't have much time, and often they're trying to do many things at once. So if meal preparation is something you need help with, let's put it on the list.

A lot of people find it helpful if their friends and neighbors pitch in to do the laundry. Someone can just drop by, pick up the hamper, and return with a basket of clean, folded linens and clothes. Right now you're getting by just throwing in a load now and then. But the time and energy it takes you to sort, move a load from the washer to the dryer, then fold, adds up. Maybe it's just an hour every few days, but wouldn't it be nice to have an extra hour just to rest, or to sit with your husband and enjoy his company?

You might want help caring for your dog. You could ask friends to walk him, or you could ask friends to be with your husband while you get out for a little while to enjoy some fresh air, a little exercise, and a break. Pets can be really good support at a time like this.

Your friends can also help run errands. It's easy enough for them to pick something up while they're out, and they'd be happy to do it. All you need to do is let them know. Some ideas include help with grocery shopping, picking up medications, or other errands.

There will still be some things you need to do—or want to do—outside the house. So you can also ask if anyone would feel comfortable staying with your husband while you're out. The hospice volunteer comes for four hours, once a week. And that may be enough, but sometimes being out of the house can give you a much-needed break. Maybe you'd like to go get your hair done, or go to church, or do something else that will help you feel refreshed. It's important to do those things. Some people feel guilty if they're not home all the time, caring for their loved one. But if you can make some time to care for yourself as well, you won't be as tired, and the time you spend with him will be better.

How to Organize This Help

Once word gets out, people will begin to contact you, offering to help. Let them know what's on your list. People will choose what they'd like to do. Some people like to cook, others will be happy to help with laundry. Someone might be happy to mow your lawn. Keep a list of all the people who have offered to help, with their phone numbers and addresses. Make note of what they're offering to do.

There will also be people who say, "If you need anything, call me, no matter what time—day or night." Make a list of these people, with their phone numbers, and keep the list in a handy place, maybe taped to the refrigerator, or some other place where you can find it in an emergency. If someone offers that, they really do mean it. That's what good friends do for one another.

When one of your more organized friends offers to help, ask if she would be willing to coordinate food. Tell her what your husband is eating, and what you'd like to eat, too. When people offer to bring food, ask them to contact the friend who's coordinating this. The coordinator can then let people know what foods you need, and when you need them. This way you don't end up with a dozen people all showing up on your doorstep at once, each bearing a pot of chicken soup. Instead, food you want to eat will be delivered on a regular basis, not all at once. When the food arrives, mark the date and the person's name on a piece of masking tape, and attach it to the dish. This way you don't have to remember how old things are, and what dish belongs to whom.

One good resource to be aware of is "Lotsa Helping Hands." It's a free Internet service that allows you to create a private Web site that you, and the people who are helping you, can access. It allows you to post your needs, and your friends, neighbors, church members, and anyone you've given password access to can log onto your site, see what you need and when you need it, and sign up.

This service also allows you to post updates on how you're both doing. This is especially helpful when a change occurs. Rather than having to call a lot of people, or having to repeat the story over and over, you can just post an update on your site and your friends can read it.

When to Seek Extra Caregiving Help

You'll want to consider asking for extra help when your husband is close to passing. At that time, it's likely that he'll need help around the clock. To have friends in the home who can help turn him, and help with other care, will give you time to rest, and time just to sit beside him, to hold his hand, to be with him as his wife. That's important.

Remember, when you ask people to help, you give them something, too—you give them that wonderful feeling of having done something that will make someone else's life better.

Relationships are all there is. Everything in the universe only exists because it is in relationship to something else. Nothing exists in isolation. We have to stop pretending we are individuals and can go it alone.

—Margaret Wheatley

ORGANIZING VOLUNTEER HELP

Make a list of tasks you need help with. Tasks might include:

- Laundry
- Meal coordination
- Cooking
- Grocery shopping and errand running
- Respite
- Walking your dog—or having someone stay with your loved one while you enjoy a walk with your dog
- Yard care
- Housekeeping

Keep a list of names with phone numbers and addresses of people who have volunteered to help. Note what each person is offering to do. Keep the list in an easily accessible place, such as on the refrigerator door.

Keep another list of names and phone numbers of people who have offered to help in an emergency, day or night. Keep that in an easy-to-find location, too.

Allow time to instruct volunteers and answer their questions. Once they are familiar with your needs and how tasks need to be done, they can save you considerable time and provide a lot of help.

Consider utilizing "Lotsa Helping Hands" to manage volunteer support. See "Appendix A: Additional Resources" (page 210).

Recognize the need for caregiver self-care and create opportunities for rest and naps.

Explore hospice support options, including nurse's aides, housekeeping support, and volunteers.

Arrange for extra support for the final days.

❧How Can I Keep Him Safe?❧

Understanding and Reducing Risks for Both the Individual and the Caregiver

Joe and Myrna

"WHAT WORRIES ME MOST IS THE FEAR THAT he'll fall," Myrna confesses as she turns to her husband, Joe, sitting beside her on their couch. "You're not as steady as you used to be."

Joe pats her hand. "I'm not going to fall."

"You might. And what will we do? I'm not strong enough to help you up."

"It's not going to happen, so don't worry."

"It might," I interject, to Joe's dismay. "But there are a lot of things we can do that might prevent a fall—or other kinds of injury—from happening. It sounds like this is a good time to talk about this, since it worries you."

"Please, I'd like to hear," Myrna says. "Joe may not worry about a fall, but I do."

"The first thing we need to do is recognize that some of this might be difficult for you, Joe. You're used to being independent. But I suspect you've noticed that your legs aren't as strong as they used to be. So the goal, I think, would be to keep you as independent and active as possible, while keeping you safe. Does that sound like what you'd like to work toward?"

"Emphasis on the active and independent part," Joe says.

"We'll do that. Let's start by considering some adaptations, based on your capabilities. We'll also want to look at preventing other kinds of injury, for both you and Myrna. Caregiving is a very physical job. We need to teach Myrna some safety tips as well, so she's not injured."

Joe's expression softens. "That's what worries me," he confesses. "Hurting Myrna. I'm afraid she'll try to help me and hurt herself."

"Then maybe listen to how we can keep you safe," Myrna admonishes. "I worry—" her voice catches. "I worry that you're going to fall and really hurt yourself."

He takes her in his arms. "I'm so sorry . . . I don't mean to worry you like that."

RECOGNIZING THE RISK

The key to preventing a fall will be your own awareness. All of us— Myrna, me, the other nurses—can watch to see how your strength holds up and encourage you to not push beyond what we think is safe, but it will be up to you to make choices about what adaptations you use, and what limits you set for yourself.

And as you've recognized, you're not the only one at risk. We need to look at ways to keep your wife safe, too. If you fall, Myrna's first impulse will be to try to catch you, or slow your fall. If that happens, it's quite likely that she'll fall, too. So the best way to keep you both safe is to be aware of the risks and take some precautions. It's important for you to continue to be as active and independent as possible, so let's look at ways to do that while improving your safety.

ADAPTING THE HOME

Let's start with your capabilities now, and look ahead at some of the adaptations you might consider later.

The first thing I'd recommend is that you create a comfortable living arrangement on the main floor. Even with adaptive devices like a cane or a walker, you won't be safe going up and down stairs. You could consider a motorized stair lift or "stair chair" as they're sometimes called, but they're expensive. You'd need to be able to safely ride one, and have a wheelchair, a walker, or some other adaptive device available at the top and bottom of the stairs. For your needs, they're probably not practical, so your best bet would be to settle on the main floor, where most of the activity takes place.

You could set up a bed in the living area for use throughout the day to conserve energy for both of you. It will provide a comfortable place for you to rest, Joe, while still being in the midst of activity, near Myrna, and with your other loved ones as they visit. You can use your couch, or hospice can bring in a hospital bed. The advantage of a hospital bed is that it adjusts, so you can sit up as well as lie down.

You can also use your recliner. You might consider asking a friend to help place a wooden block or some kind of riser to elevate it to a height that's comfortable for you to get up from.

I'd also recommend picking up all the throw rugs. When we're tired, or not as strong, we tend not to lift our feet as much when we walk, so we're more likely to trip on uneven surfaces, like throw rugs.

To conserve energy, I'd recommend a bath bench. This allows you to safely get in and out of the tub, and sit while you shower. You can find new bath benches at medical supply stores, or used ones through craigslist. You'll probably also want to get a toilet riser. It's a seat that fits over the toilet, making the seat higher. It has handrails you can use to help yourself down and up again. A lot of people find them very helpful.

You might also consider installing safety bars in the bathroom. You'll need to decide if the cost of installation is worthwhile for the time you'll be using them. It's likely that in a few months you'll no longer be able to get around in the bathroom. But if Myrna is planning to stay in the house and she'll benefit from them, too, it might be worthwhile to get them installed now.

You might also want to plug in nightlights throughout the house. Given the medications you take to help you sleep, you might feel a little groggy when you wake up at night, and the extra light will help you navigate without banging into things. Better yet, to avoid having to walk to the bathroom when you're groggy, you could keep a urinal or a bedside commode next to the bed.

It's important to make sure your smoke alarm batteries are working. Because you're not able to move as quickly as you used to, if you do have a fire, you'll want all the warning you can get.

Another handy tool is a portable monitor or walkie-talkies. Also, some cordless phones have multiple handsets and can be used as an intercom.

By using some kind of intercom or monitor, you can be in one room and Myrna can be in another, and you'll be able to hear each other.

You can find monitors in stores that sell baby items. The advantage of a monitor is that Myrna can hear what's happening in the room at all times, without you having to push a button to talk or get her attention. For example, if you did fall, she would hear you. The disadvantage is that the communication is one-way. Myrna can hear you, but she has to come to you to reply. Intercoms are two-way, but you have to push a button to talk.

MAXIMIZING MOBILITY

To keep you as active and mobile as possible, we have adaptive devices, things like walkers, four-point canes, and wheelchairs. These can give you extra stability and conserve your energy for the things that matter most to you.

I know it's not easy to think about using these things. But you've both shared that you're afraid of what a fall could mean, for each of you. And I suspect, Joe, that it can sometimes be tiring for you to get around. Using mobility tools is a good way to decrease your risks, conserve your energy, increase your mobility, and give you both more peace of mind.

If, in the future, you find you need help getting up or transferring from the bed to a wheelchair, there are some other tools and techniques we can offer. The nurse's aide or a physical therapist can show you these transfer techniques so you both stay safe.

RECOGNIZING WHEN YOU NEED HELP

It's going to be hard for you to recognize when you need the extra help, or devices like a cane, walker, or wheelchair. Losing independence is one of the biggest challenges people face. The best advice I can offer is to listen to your body. Do your legs feel a bit shaky when you walk? Is it becoming difficult to get up from a chair? Do you need to hold on to things when you walk? Are you steady when you walk? If not, it's probably time to start using some of these tools.

Most importantly, listen to your wife. Listen when she shares her fears and worries. And share your worries with her, too. You're on this journey together.

Preventing Other Problems

We should also talk about the other risks of decreased mobility, things you might not have thought about. But here, too, with awareness and a few preventive measures, you can avoid these problems.

Preventing Pressure Wounds

If you spend a lot of time sitting or lying down, you face the risk of a pressure wound, commonly called a bedsore. Basically, the tissues in our body are nourished by the nutrients and oxygen carried in the bloodstream. Think of blood vessels as being like straws. If we compress them, less fluid can pass through. This is especially true of bony pressure points, like our tailbone, hips, and heels. And if we stay in one position for a long period, the tissues don't get the oxygen and nutrients they need, and damage occurs *on the inside*.

At first, there'll be no sign of damage. But late in the process, the skin in that area will turn a dusky red, and remain red, even after the pressure is relieved. The only way to prevent it from becoming worse is to keep pressure off that area and let it heal. Otherwise, the damage will continue, and suddenly a wound will open up through our skin and our favorite position will become painful, even intolerable.

But remember, you can prevent pressure wounds. To do that, you'll want to change positions at least every two hours. Most of us get some kind of cue when we've been sitting too long. Our bottom, hips, or heels go numb, or become sore, and so we shift. But as we age—and sometimes as a result of medication we're taking, or if we've had chemotherapy—we don't always sense when we're sore or numb.

So note how long you sit or lie in one position. Set a timer if you need to, and every two hours, change positions. You can tip a little to one side or the other. Use pillows as props—anything that works for you.

Just keep good circulation flowing, and you won't develop a pressure wound.

Preventing Choking

As the body weakens, another risk is the potential for choking. But again, awareness of what's causing the risks, and what to do about them, can prevent this problem.

One cause relates to how you're eating and drinking. With decreased mobility, it's likely that you'll be doing more eating or drinking while reclined in bed or in a chair. In that position, you face an increased risk of choking. That's easy enough to change. You just raise the head of the bed or recliner, and sit up to eat or drink.

But there's another risk to be aware of. For some people, the ability to swallow diminishes with progressive illness, and you may not, at least initially, be aware of it. So, to reduce your risk, take smaller bites. Chew your food well. Always eat or drink sitting up.

If you do notice a change in your ability to swallow, talk with us. We'll help you to find an adaptation that works for you. That may be having someone with you when you eat or drink. For some people, just being reminded to swallow is enough. For others, changing the temperature or texture of the food or drink helps. We have lots of tools, so let us know if swallowing becomes a problem.

Preventing Burns

If you use an electric heating pad, you run the risk of a burn, even at a low setting. With illness, age, and some treatments like radiation and chemotherapy, people may lose some of the sensitivity in their skin. Also, you may be sleeping more, and you might fall asleep on a heating pad.

To safely use an electric heating pad, set it on low, but don't place it on the skin. Instead, set a timer for ten to fifteen minutes and let it heat up. Then unplug it and place it on the affected area. Cover it with a dry towel to help hold in the heat, and leave it in place. When it cools off, take it off, reheat it, and replace it as often as you need to.

Caregiver Safety

When one partner is no longer able to do what he used to, the other partner often takes on additional tasks. This can be tiring. It will likely involve a lot more physical activity than she's used to.

As a caregiver, one thing you'll want to do is remember to lift with your legs and not your back. When you lift anything, no matter how light it is, don't bend over. Squat instead. Keep your back straight and your head up. Take hold of the object and straighten your legs. That's how you lift safely. If the object is too heavy, call someone to help—a neighbor perhaps. Don't try to lift something heavy by yourself.

Also, you might be tempted to retrieve things from high places that you can't safely reach. Keep a sturdy step stool handy and remember to use it. You could also use an extension gripper device, or simply move the things you use most often to lower shelves.

Most important, if Joe does fall, don't try to catch him. That's easier said than done. Our first instinct when someone's falling is to help. If you do try to help, it's likely you'll fall, too. So if he goes down, try to not break his fall, then call us. We'll help you figure out if he's hurt.

If he's not hurt, and feels he can get up with a little help, you could place a sturdy chair beside him for him to push up from. If he needs more help than that, we can call the nonemergency number for the local fire department. Most fire departments offer a service called a Fireman's Assist. They'll come to the home and help him up.

Of course, the best solution is for him to use the tools and adaptations we're talking about, use good judgment, stay safe, and not fall in the first place. Yes, his strength and energy level will likely decline, but there are ways to keep both of you safe, as active as possible, and energetic as possible to enjoy the things that matter most to you.

Nothing in life is to be feared. It is only to be understood.

—Marie Curie

Safety Tips
Preventing Falls

- Arrange to live on the main floor and eliminate the need to climb stairs.
- Create a comfortable environment in a central location to minimize movement.
- Place a sturdy table with frequently needed objects within easy reach.
- Ask a physical therapist to evaluate the height of your recliner or favorite chair. In many cases, the chair can be placed on a wooden block, raising the height and making it easier for you to get up.
- Remove throw rugs.
- Keep floors free of clutter and hallways clear.
- Use nightlights.
- Use adaptive devices, like a four-point cane, a walker, or a wheelchair for added stability and energy conservation.
- Use adaptive devices in the bathroom, including a bath bench and toilet riser.
- For longer-term arrangements, consider installing grab bars in the bathroom.
- Use a urinal or bedside commode at night, or whenever you have decreased mobility.
- Use a monitor or intercom to communicate between rooms.
- Make sure that smoke detectors are working properly.

Preventing Pressure Wounds

- Reposition yourself every two hours, minimum—more often if you are especially thin or your skin is reddened. Consider setting a timer as a reminder.
- Use pillows for propping yourself up.
- Ask someone to examine your skin frequently for redness. If an area remains a dusky red, keep pressure off that area until the redness resolves. Common areas for pressure wounds include the hips, tailbone, and heels. For more information about checking for

pressure wounds, see "How Do I Bring the Bathroom to Him?" (page 85).

Preventing Choking

- Always eat or drink in an upright position.
- Take small bites.
- Chew well.
- If problems with swallowing occur, talk with your health care provider or hospice team.

Preventing Burns

- If you use an electric heating pad, preheat it; then turn it off and unplug it before placing it on your skin.
- If you smoke, do so carefully, and make sure that someone is with you to ensure that you don't fall asleep with a lit cigarette.
- If you have oxygen in the home, don't use it near any open flames (cigarettes, candles, fires in fireplaces, a gas stove, a woodstove, etc.).

Preventing Back and Other Injuries for Caregivers

- For all lifting, lift with the legs, not the back. When lifting, do not bend over. Squat with the back straight and the head up. Take hold of the object and straighten the legs to lift. Ask a nurse, a nurse's aide, or a physical therapist to help you learn this technique.
- Keep a sturdy step stool handy to reach items on high shelves.
- Keep items you use most often within easy reach.
- Arrange a session with a nurse's aide or a physical therapist to learn safe ways to help your loved one pivot from a bed to a wheelchair or bedside commode.
- Do not attempt to stop someone from falling.

How Do I Bring the Bathroom to Him?

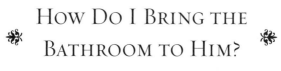

Options for Toileting and Bathing

Jack and Molly

"It's getting pretty difficult for him to get around in the bathroom," Molly says, gripping her coffee mug. "Until now we've been managing with the bath bench and a toilet riser. It's not always easy. There's not a lot of room in there for his walker, and I don't think a wheelchair will fit. He's getting weaker. He's not able to bear his weight for long. I'm afraid his legs might buckle and take both of us down. I try to help him, but it's just not safe anymore." She sighs. "What are we going to do?"

"You're wise to recognize that it's not safe for you to continue to try to help Jack move around in the bathroom. If he's having difficulty bearing his weight, a fall could hurt you both. So at this point, we need to figure out how he can be cared for within these limitations.

"You've already set a bed up in the living room, so that will help. With the bed where everyone spends most of the day, he's still in the midst of things, and doesn't have to move around as much. And as long as he's able to bear some of his weight, you can still help him pivot from a bed to a wheelchair, as the nurse's aide showed you.

"But we need to make some adaptations for bathing and toileting. Let's talk about bathing first. We can have the nurse's aide come to the house a few times a week to give him a bath. Given all that you have to do, I'd recommend that help."

"Let's do that. But I think I should know how to give a basic bed bath, just in case he needs one between the aide's visits," Molly says.

How to Give a Bed Bath and Inspect the Skin for Pressure Wounds

Bed baths are actually pretty easy to give, and he can help as much as he's able. To give him a bed bath, you'll want to gather your supplies: a small garbage bag—those plastic bags you get at the grocery store work well—two or three towels; a couple of washcloths; a few disposable cloths, like baby wipes; a basin with warm water—test it to make sure it's not too hot—and a little no-rinse soap. You don't need much, just a little. If you don't have no-rinse soap, you'll need a second basin with warm water and a few extra washcloths for rinsing.

You can also smooth lotion on his skin as you give the bath. One handy trick is to put the lotion bottle in the bathwater to warm it. That way the lotion isn't cold on his skin.

Start by creating some privacy. Close the drapes or blinds. If other people are in the house, close the door to the room, or ask for privacy if you can't close off the room. To keep him from becoming chilled during the bath, leave him covered with the blankets until you're ready to wash each area.

Start with his face. Wet the washcloth in the soapy water and gently wipe his eyes first, then the rest of his face. The idea is that at the beginning, the washcloth is the cleanest, so we start with the face. After you wipe his skin with the cloth from the soapy water, dip another washcloth into your rinse water and wipe the area a couple of times. If you have no-rinse soap, skip the rinse step. After you wash and rinse an area, pat him dry with a towel, and apply lotion.

Next, ease the covers toward the center of his chest, exposing one arm and half of his torso. Wash this half of his chest and his arm. Rinse, dry, apply lotion, then cover him back up. Next, ease aside the covers over his leg. Wash, rinse, dry, apply lotion, and replace the covers.

Next, uncover his groin area. You'll want to use a disposable cloth here. Wash his groin, then throw the cloth away. If you need to keep washing that area, get a fresh disposable cloth each time. You don't want to get your wash water dirty with what you've washed this area of his skin. After you dry that area, have him roll to his side. Wash his bottom with disposable cloths, then rinse, dry, and apply lotion. Then, with him still on his side, using the regular washcloth, wash his back; then dry that area and apply lotion.

Before you have him roll back onto his back, take a close look at his skin. The backside is especially vulnerable to pressure wounds, commonly called bedsores. Look for reddened areas, especially at the tailbone, hips, or other bony areas, like the spine. If you see an area that's red, gently press your finger against that red area. It should turn pale momentarily, then the color should return. If it doesn't turn pale, but remains red, especially a dusky red, call us. That's the beginning of a pressure wound. We'll give you instructions on what to do.

After you finish washing, applying lotion, and inspecting his back and bottom, help him roll onto his back again, cover him up, and move to the other side, washing first his arm and torso, and then his leg and hip. You'll finish by washing, rinsing, drying, and applying lotion to his feet. As you wash the feet, be sure to inspect the heels. They're also vulnerable to pressure wounds.

WHY AM I USING REGULAR WASHCLOTHS IN ONE PLACE AND DISPOSABLE CLOTHS IN ANOTHER?

You're using the regular washcloths only in areas with normal skin bacteria. The groin and rectal area likely have traces of urine or fecal matter, which you don't want to introduce to the water. You can use baby wipes, if you like. When washing these areas, dip the clean, disposable cloth in the wash water; wipe; and then throw this cloth out. Don't put a soiled, disposable cloth from the groin or rectal area back into the clean water. Use as many disposable cloths as you need to finish the job.

IS THERE AN EASY WAY TO MANAGE ALL THIS LAUNDRY?

You might want to keep a good stock of linens so that you don't have to do laundry as often. Consider a visit to a thrift shop to buy some extra washcloths and towels. Another time-saver would be to have a special basket or hamper just for washcloths and towels. When you're running low, just throw that load in the washer. This way you don't have to sort all the other laundry just for this linen. When it's dry, just pile it into a basket. You don't need to fold it. Just pull what you need from there. If you're caring for someone with respiratory problems, it's a good idea to use unscented laundry soap and avoid scented fabric softeners.

What about Brushing His Teeth?

You'll want to bring supplies to him to brush his teeth. In addition to the toothbrush and toothpaste, he'll need a glass of water, a small basin to spit in, and a towel to wipe his mouth. It doesn't have to be a fancy basin. You can use a plastic container or margarine dish. It just needs to be large enough so it's easy for him to spit into.

What If He Can't Get to the Toilet?

To urinate, he can use a urinal. After he's finished, you just pour the urine in the toilet. Then pour some water into the urinal, swish it around, and pour that into the toilet as well. Every few days you might want to add a little vinegar to the rinse water to clean the urinal more thoroughly.

When he needs to have a bowel movement, he'll use a bedside commode. It's a sturdy seat with handholds and a basin below the seat. Close the drapes or blinds. Then, using the technique the nurse's aide showed you, he can simply swing his legs to the floor and pivot onto the seat. You'll want to have the seat cover up and his pajamas down before he pivots.

Leave toilet tissue or baby wipes within easy reach. One tip: While toilet tissue certainly works, baby wipes will speed the cleanup. Just be sure to drop them in a wastebasket lined with a disposable garbage bag, not the commode, since they can't be flushed down the toilet.

Offer to step out of the room to provide some privacy. He can call you when he's finished. Some people place a baby monitor in the room, so if they're out of voice range they can still hear their loved one.

When he finishes and is back in bed, simply lift the basin and pour the contents into the toilet. To clean it, add water and a little toilet-bowl cleaner, and wash it out with a toilet brush. Pour the wash water into the toilet and flush.

You might also consider having air freshener handy, though for people with respiratory problems, you'll want to avoid scented products.

How Do We Manage Disposable Underwear?

There may come a time when he's not able to pivot to the bedside commode, or when he might not be aware that he's emptied his bladder or bowels. If that happens, he'll need to use disposable underwear. Some people call them diapers, but I prefer to call them disposable underwear.

If he needs to use disposable underwear, you'll want to keep some supplies on hand: a basin, disposable wipes, disposable latex gloves for you, disposable underwear, and some small plastic garbage bags.

To change the underwear, put on gloves and remove the soiled underwear, placing it in the plastic bag. To clean him, use the same technique you used with the bed bath to wash his groin and bottom, placing only clean, disposable wipes in the water. If you use premoistened wipes, you might be able to get by without the wash water, but for larger clean-ups, using soapy water can speed the process.

After wiping, drop the soiled disposable cloths in the plastic garbage bag. When you finish cleaning him, throw your gloves in the bag, too. Knot the top of the bag and throw it away. By tying up the bag, you'll help contain odors. Put on fresh disposable underwear, then finish by washing your hands.

The best way to learn how to get the underwear on and off is to have us show you. It's actually not too difficult. So if he does need disposable underwear, ask the nurse's aide or one of us nurses to show you how.

How Can I Make This Easier for Him to Accept?

For him, this is one more loss of independence, and may feel like a loss of dignity. But, truthfully, it happens to nearly everyone at some point in this journey. We leave the world much the way we enter it—dependent on others.

Someday I, too, will probably need someone to help me clean up. If someone I'm caring for is really embarrassed, I'll share that with them. It helps put it into perspective. One other idea would be to tell him that if your positions were reversed, and you were the one needing help, that he'd be doing this for you.

Although the world is full of suffering, it is also full of the overcoming of it.

—Helen Keller

Personal Care Supplies

Organizing Supplies

- Consider purchasing additional washcloths and towels, either new or secondhand. Reserve a separate laundry hamper for them, reducing the need for sorting and minimizing the frequency of washing. After washing, place unfolded towels and cloths in a basket near where they'll be used.
- Consider purchasing a supply of oversized T-shirts and drawstring pajama bottoms. For ease in dressing, consider cutting the T-shirts up the back, leaving the neck intact. This may be helpful later on, if your loved one needs total care and is unable to get out of bed.
- Organize disposable underwear supplies together in a washbasin.
- Organize bed bath supplies in a second basin.

Bed Bath Supplies

- One large basin for washing
- Second large basin for rinsing, if no-rinse soap is not available

- No-rinse or liquid soap (use unscented soap if the person has respiratory problems)
- Lotion
- Disposable wipes
- Washcloths
- Several towels
- Clean clothes to wear after the bath
- Basket or hamper for used towels and washcloths
- Small garbage bag (used plastic grocery bags work well)

Disposable Underwear Supplies

- One large basin
- Disposable wipes or premoistened wipes
- No-rinse soap (if using regular soap, add a second basin for rinse water)
- Small plastic garbage bags (used plastic grocery bags work well)
- Disposable latex gloves, sized for caregivers
- Disposable underwear, properly sized (too big is better than too small)
- Air freshener spray

Other Personal Care Supplies

- Small basin for tooth brushing
- Nonbreakable glass or cup
- Toothbrush
- Toothpaste
- Hand towel
- Electric shaver
- Liquid toilet-bowl cleaner and bowl brush to clean the bedside commode basin
- Vinegar for rinsing the urinal

❋ I Don't Know What to Say... ❋

Insights to Achieve a Meaningful Visit

Hanna

"Why are they sending me a get well card?" asks Hanna, her brows wrinkling as she gazes up from the bed. "They know I'm not going to get well."

I hesitate, trying to find an answer. "Sometimes people just don't know what to say. In our culture, it's as if we don't want to acknowledge that we die. So we sweep it under the rug. Out of sight, out of mind."

She picks up the card and reads, "Here's hoping you'll be kicking up your heels again soon! Wishing you a speedy recovery..." She frowns. Then a light flashes in her eyes. "You know, if I were up to kicking up my heels again, I'd start a business making greeting cards for a time like this."

"What would the cards say?"

"Lots of things. Things I'd like to talk with my friends about. Things I wish they could understand. Things I wish they could help *me* understand."

"Sounds like a worthwhile endeavor."

She nods. "Hand me that pad of paper, will you? I'm going to write this down. Maybe somebody else will do it. Better yet, will you write it down? My handwriting isn't so good these days."

I sit and perch the pad on my lap.

"You know, it's not just greeting cards," she says. "Cards are just where you start. What I really wish is that when people come to visit we could have a really meaningful conversation."

"That would be nice."

"It doesn't have to be sad and gloomy, either. I still laugh. Even with all this. Laughing is good. You can talk about meaning and hope and all those things, and still laugh."

I smile and scribble a note. *Laugh with me.*

"People don't understand that there's still hope—not for a cure, but for something else, a good day, a good visit with a friend, a little sunshine . . . There's hope for bigger things, too, like hope for quality time with the people I love, hope for closure, for knowing that my kids will be okay when I'm gone, that I've left them with the ability to live a meaningful life. And, yes, when the end does come, I hope for peace. Every day there's still something to hope for. I don't think they get that.

"And another thing . . . Sometimes people just come in and tell me what they think. They don't really want to hear what I think, or what worries me, or what I hope for. They just say things like, 'You're going to beat this.' " She frowns. "Like *that's* helpful. Or another one: 'Doctors are wrong all the time. You're going to be fine.' " She sighs. "How helpful is it to tell me my doctor is wrong? That I should question all the really difficult decisions I've made? How helpful is it to tell me that my being sick, that my facing death is all some mistake?

"Why can't we talk about what our friendship—what the life we share together—means? Why can't they look at me and not turn away, or wince because I have no hair? Why can't they look at me and acknowledge the courage it takes to walk down this road, to make these choices, to believe in myself, to live the best I can, for however long I can?"

Then, in a voice barely above a whisper, she adds, "Why can't they tell me I have courage? That I have strength? Even though I'm sick and don't have long to live, why can't they tell me I have value? That what I leave behind—the time we've spent together—has value?"

She reaches for my hand and squeezes. Then she leans against me. I hold her. For a long time she sobs. Then she straightens and wipes her eyes. "Pick up that pad of paper again, will you? I have something to say."

A real friend is one who walks in when the rest of the world walks out.
—Walter Winchell

SUGGESTIONS FOR MEANINGFUL COMMUNICATION

- Laugh with me.
- Talk with me about the times we shared, and what these times mean to you.
- Talk with me about what you've learned from me and from the journey I'm taking, a journey that someday you, too, will take.
- Talk with me about our friends. Include me by sharing news about gatherings or activities in which I can no longer participate.
- When possible, bring these gatherings or activities to me.
- Choose cards with themes of friendship, laughter, or courage.
- Respect that I may be tired and need to rest. Visit me more frequently, but for short periods of time.
- Respect that I have done the best I could to make good decisions with a team of people I trust. Support me by honoring these choices.
- Find a way to feel comfortable with silence, with just sitting beside me or holding my hand. I may not always feel like talking, and having a friend just be with me is sometimes a great comfort.
- Listen. Support me while I find my own answers to questions about meaning, peace, and other issues. Recognize that what's right for you may not be what's right for me.
- If I tell you what I'm afraid of, or what worries me, please just listen. Allow me to talk. Sometimes just talking about something helps me to work through it. In most cases, you won't be able to "fix" it, but you can listen, and that will help a lot.
- Accept that when my time is very near, I will have very little energy, and may want only family or very close friends around me.
- Most important, know that time is short. We go though life with too much small talk. If there are important, meaningful things that you want to say to me, say them now. There will never be a better time.

Words to Try

When You Think You Want to Say:	Try This Instead:
Dad, you are going to be just fine	Dad, are there some things that worry you?
Don't talk like that! You can beat this!	It must be hard to come to terms with all this.
I can't see how anyone can help.	We will be there for you, always.
I just can't talk about this.	I am feeling a little overwhelmed right now. Can we take this up later tonight?
What do the doctors know? You might live forever.	Do you think the doctors are right? How does it seem to you?
Please don't give up. I need you here.	I need you here. I will miss you terribly. But we will get through somehow.
There has to be something more to do.	Let's be sure we get the best of medical treatments, but let's be together when we have done all we can.
Don't be glum. You will get well.	It must be hard. Can I just sit with you for a while?

From *Handbook for Mortals,* Joanne Lynn, M.D. and Joan Harrold, M.D. By Permission of Oxford University Press, Inc.

❈ He Doesn't Want to Eat . . . ❈

Understanding and Adapting to a Changing Appetite
Ideas for Adapting Meal Schedules for
People with Memory Impairment
Suggestions for Easy-to-Digest Foods and Beverages

Robert and Susan

"HE DOESN'T EAT MUCH," SUSAN SAYS, as she sits beside her father in his living room.

I glance at Robert, at his sunken cheeks, at the plaid cotton shirt that hangs on his gaunt frame, at the caring gaze he directs at his daughter.

"You've got to eat," she says, clutching her notepad, which chronicles each day's activity: what time he got up, what medicines he took, what he ate. "It's the only way you're going to keep up your strength."

When Susan steps out of the room, I perform a brief physical exam and ask Robert a few questions. I learn that he has no sore throat, no difficulty swallowing, no nausea or vomiting, no constipation, no depression, no shortness of breath when eating, no pain—nothing that could account for a decrease in appetite and could be treated. The medication he's been taking for the past three months to stimulate his appetite worked well at first. But now, as his disease progresses, it's no longer effective.

"I just can't eat," Robert confides. "I want to. She goes to so much trouble to make me the kind of foods I used to love. And when I can't eat them, she goes back into the kitchen and makes me these protein shakes." His eyes mist with tears. "I try. For her, I try. But I just can't eat more than a few bites. If I do, I feel nauseous.

"Having her around these past few months has been wonderful, but my body is just giving out." He reaches for my hand. "Can you help me explain this to her? I've tried, but . . . I don't know how. It's so hard.

She looks at me with such hope. She thinks that if I eat, then at least I won't get worse."

Moments later, Susan returns and settles beside her father. "So how's he doing?"

"How do you feel he's doing?" I ask gently.

She turns to her father. "Well, he seems a bit weaker, and he's sleeping more. He's getting thinner. If he could just eat more, I think he'd be doing much better." She turns to me. "What if we increase the medicine he takes to improve his appetite? Would that help?"

"The medicine he's been taking to improve his appetite usually works only for a little while. I also checked to see if there might be another cause for his declining appetite—something we could treat."

"And?"

"We found no treatable cause. Unfortunately, loss of appetite is part of the process."

Susan frowns. "There must be something we can do . . ."

"Do you remember a time when you didn't feel well, when you just didn't feel like eating much? Maybe just toast, a little soup, some juice. That's your body's way of taking care of itself, its way of sending signals about what it needs, what it can do, and what it can't do. When we're sick, our body uses its energy to deal with what's causing it harm. It hasn't got the energy to digest complex foods. You may have noticed that when your dad got sick he didn't want to eat much meat, and then he didn't want to eat any meat at all. That was his body saying, 'I can't digest this.' If he tried, if he forced himself to eat, because he thought he needed to, or wanted to for you, then he probably felt nauseous, and maybe even vomited."

Susan turns to her dad. "Is that true?"

He gazes at her, then slowly nods.

"When we're sick," I add, "we generally can't eat a full meal. It's just too much at once, so we eat smaller meals or snacks, choosing more easily digested foods, like puddings, mashed potatoes, juice—things like that."

"But he's got to eat," she implores. "If he doesn't eat . . . If he doesn't eat, he'll die."

Robert takes hold of his daughter's hand.

"When we eat," I say, "everything is normal. From the time we're born, and throughout our lives, sharing food is an act of love. When we gather with our family, with our friends, we share meals. It's how we celebrate. It's how we nurture one another. And here you are, with love for your father, wanting to take care of him. You make these wonderful meals and high-nutrition shakes, putting all your love and care into each of them. If he eats, then everything will be all right. If he eats, everything is normal. If he eats, he won't die . . ."

Susan closes her eyes and tears begin to stream down her face. She buries her face in her hands and leans against her dad. "I don't want you to die!"

Robert draws Susan into his arms. Tears flow down his cheeks as well.

"All your life your dad's been there for you. And if he could, he'd stay with you forever."

Susan burrows closer into Robert's arms. For a long time he holds her, rocking her gently, his face nuzzled in her hair.

"I love you, Daddy," she whispers.

"I know, sweetheart. I love you too, so very much . . . and I wish, more than anything, that I could change this."

"I don't want you to feel sick when you eat. And I don't want you to eat if you don't want to, or if you can't."

Robert brushes his thumb against Susan's cheek, wiping away a tear. "Have I told you what having you here these past months has meant to me? You've done more for me than any medicine, or any steak dinner ever could have."

"I'm so glad I came, to be with you now . . . I love you, Daddy. I love you."

I sit quietly. This is their moment. When they turn to me again I share some ideas. "There are some things you can do, some ways to adjust to a decreasing appetite that might be helpful," I offer gently. "You can make your dad snacks, easily digested foods, things he can eat, and keep a supply of them in the refrigerator. In general, it's easier to digest carbohydrates and simple proteins. I'll leave you a list of ideas for foods you might want to try.

"When he does feel like eating, put a little in a small bowl or on a small plate, just a few bites. If he wants more, you can get it, but sometimes just being offered a small amount makes it feel less overwhelming.

"You can also keep a small glass—just a few ounces—of his favorite nutrition drink or juice beside him throughout the day, so if he feels like a sip now and then, it's there. Every hour or so, replace it with a fresh glass, so you don't risk spoilage.

"The other thing you can do, and maybe the most important thing, is let him know it's okay for him not to eat, that he's not disappointing you, or letting you down. Let him know you accept that just being with him is enough."

Susan turns to her father. "I don't want you to feel that you have to do something just for me. You don't need to fight just for me. And you don't have to force yourself to eat. Whatever time we have now is a gift . . ."

Elizabeth and Her Family

"It's becoming harder and harder to get her to eat," says Rhonda, Elizabeth's caregiver.

Tina, Elizabeth's daughter, adds, "We try to tell her she needs to eat, but I don't think she understands. It's the Alzheimer's. She doesn't remember that she needs to eat. She'll say she just ate and isn't hungry, or that she's not hungry and will wait to have dinner with my father when he comes home. My father's been dead for ten years."

"How do you and your brothers feel about your mother not eating much?"

"Well, we don't want to force her, but she doesn't understand. We don't want to starve her to death."

"How active is Elizabeth? Does she sleep most of the time?"

"Yes," Rhonda answers. "And it's getting harder to wake her in the morning at breakfast time. When I try to feed her, she nods off. It's that way at lunch and dinner time, too."

"Is there a reason why she needs to eat at a certain time?"

"We give her medicine four times a day," Rhonda says. "We give the medicine with meals, and a snack at bedtime, so she's not taking all those pills on an empty stomach."

"Let's look at her medicine list." Together we review the list and discover that most of her medicine can be taken on an empty stomach. Only two pills need to be taken with food. I point them out, adding, "She can take these with milk, or a few crackers. That will be enough to prevent an upset stomach."

Rhonda makes a note in the caregiver log.

"Let's look at the bigger issue. You shared that your mother doesn't understand that she needs to eat. With Alzheimer's, and dementia in general, we lose our short-term memory. We may not remember when we ate, or what we ate, but we still feel hunger. We still feel thirst. We may not remember when we last slept, but we still know when we want to sleep.

"Your mother knows when she's hungry and when she's not. The confusion for her is that when she's offered a meal, when her caregivers tell her it's time to eat, she knows she *should* be hungry, but often, she's not. So she tries to understand. She can't remember, but there must be a reason, so she struggles to come up with one: Maybe she just ate, maybe she had a snack so she could eat later, with your father . . ."

"So it's her lack of appetite, not the confusion that causes her to not want to eat?" Tina asks.

"Exactly."

She turns to Rhonda. "Does this fit with what you see Mom do?"

"When we offer her meals she gets flustered," Rhonda says. "Then she tries to refuse, saying she just ate, things like that. Usually, we can persuade her to take a few bites, but she never eats a full meal anymore."

"So what do we do? How do we get Mom to eat?"

"The question, perhaps, is this: How do we deal with food in a way that's right for your mom, so she still feels honored and respected?"

"I like that approach much better. How do we do that?"

I share the reasons why the appetite declines and suggest frequent snacks of easy-to-digest foods, rather than full meals.

"She may not want to eat at regular mealtimes," I add. "But she may be hungry an hour later. When she's awake, bring in a few bites of custard, or applesauce, or a nutrition drink, and ask her how she would feel about taking a few bites. Don't ask her to eat or drink for you, or tell her that she needs to eat, or has to eat. Let it be her choice. If she's hungry, she'll eat. If she's not, she won't. If she doesn't eat, then come back an hour later, or if she goes to sleep, ask her again when she wakes up.

"Also, even if you leave food or drinks beside her, she may not remember that they're there. So with memory impairment, it's helpful to gently offer, but don't, in any way, insist."

"But what if she doesn't want to eat much?" Tina asks. "What do we do?"

"She'll eat what her body tells her it needs. As she progresses on her journey, she'll want less and less. That's her body following its natural process. To force her would be to override that natural protection and will cause her discomfort. If she eats too much, she'll feel nauseous, and may vomit."

"We don't want that. We just want to do the right thing, to take care of her . . ." Tina's voice catches. "We want her to feel loved, respected, and cared for."

One word frees us of all the weight and pain of life: That word is love.
—*Sophocles*

ADAPTATIONS FOR CHANGES IN APPETITE
Offering Food and Beverages

- Plan for meals and snacks for both the person affected by illness and the caregiver(s).

- Prepare several servings at one time. Freeze and label leftovers in one or two serving sizes for later use. (For labeling, masking tape works well. Remove tape before placing the container in the oven or microwave.)

- Once food is thawed, mark the thaw date on the tape and refrigerate it. Discard unused refrigerated food after five days, or sooner, if needed.

- Keep on hand prepared snacks, such as ready-made puddings, cookies, fruit cocktail, crackers, cheese, bread for toast, etc. For ways to tap friends/volunteers to keep the kitchen well-stocked with ready-to-eat food, see "I Can't Do This Alone . . ." (page 71).

- When purchasing ready-made foods, check nutrition labels and avoid high-sodium foods. (USRDA recommendation: less than 2,300 milligrams of sodium per day. In cases of heart or kidney disease, or high blood pressure, consult your health care provider.)

- When leaving perishable food or drinks at room temperature, refresh them every hour, or more frequently, if needed, to prevent spoilage.

- For people who experience shortness of breath or tire easily, offer food that doesn't require much chewing.

- For people with memory impairment, offer snacks frequently. It's possible they may not remember that a food or beverage is right next to them.

- Consider using straws.

- Serve food and beverages in small plates, bowls, and glasses to make everything look more like a full meal.

- When collecting used dishes and glasses, don't comment about how much or how little was consumed.

- Ask the person if she *would like* something to eat or drink. Don't say that she *needs* to eat, or *should* eat.

- Don't show disappointment if she doesn't eat. Let it be her choice, and honor that choice.

Easily Digested Foods
- Pudding
- Custard
- Mashed potatoes
- Ice cream
- Pastas in cream sauce
- Scrambled eggs
- Applesauce
- Toast
- Milkshakes or smoothies
- Nutrition drinks or Instant Breakfast
- Soups (check sodium content if canned)
- Popsicles
- Fruit juice

For Family Discussion
- Why is our loved one not eating?
- Has the health care provider ruled out treatable causes for declining appetite?
- How do we feel about our loved one's declining appetite?
- What can each of us do to support our loved one and each other? Ideas include sharing in the task of preparing meals and snacks to keep on hand, and sharing in the task of preparing meals for the caregiver.

For Loved Ones Who Live Far Away: What Can I Do?

Staying Informed and Supportive
Deciding When to Visit

Ferdinand and David

"I'll walk you out," David says. He turns to this father. "I'll be right back, Dad."

As we walk toward my car, David jams his hands in his pockets. I slow my pace, sensing that there are questions he wants to ask, questions he doesn't want his father to hear. At the car I turn to him. "How are you holding up?"

He shrugs. "Okay, I guess."

"Your dad mentioned that he talked with your brothers and sisters yesterday. How did that go?"

"Well, it's a little difficult. They don't really see what's going on."

David's siblings, though educated in the United States, all returned to the Philippines to live. Only David, the youngest, remained after graduating from college three years ago.

"When was the last time they saw your dad?"

"A couple of months ago. Most of the family flew in and stayed for a week." His gaze falls to his shoes. "They think he's still like that. Still getting around okay, still eating like he used to." He shakes his head. "They think I should be doing a lot of things differently."

On the recommendation of David's eldest brother, a doctor, the family decided that their father should come to the United States for treatment. When the treatments failed to bring about a cure and Ferdinand's needs increased, David took a leave from his high-tech job to care for their father.

"What do you tell them about how he's doing?"

"I try to tell them how things are, but it's as if they have another idea, that Dad isn't really that sick, that if I made sure he got enough to eat, got exercise, didn't sleep all day, he'd be all right.

"They call all the time, asking what Dad's doing, how much he's eating, and tell me what I should do, but . . . I don't mean to complain. I know each of them wishes they were here, taking care of him."

"Does your dad talk with them about how he's doing?"

"Sure he does, except what he tells them isn't what's really going on. He doesn't want to worry them. He always puts us kids first."

"It must be hard to be in the middle, to see how your father's doing every day, and have your family, who doesn't see it—but has the best intentions—try to manage the situation from so far away."

"And my brother's a doctor, too. He knows a lot more than I do about this kind of thing, but it's as if he can't see that Dad is declining . . . pretty fast, too."

"He's a doctor, but he's also a son. It's hard to think of our loved ones declining, especially when we're so far away. Because we're not there every day, seeing the changes, we're able to create an image of what we want, rather than what is. And we hold on to that image out of hope. We also hold that image because, being so far away, unable to be with the person we love, we feel helpless. So we spend our time thinking about how we can improve the situation. When we hear that the situation doesn't match our image, often we push even harder.

"It's difficult to accept that, no matter what we do, we can't bring about a cure for our loved one. But I think it's especially difficult if the ties are strong and we live far away."

"I wish they could see him as he is," David says.

"What has your father told you about what he wants?"

"He says he's ready to go. He's tired. He says he couldn't have asked for a better life. Did you know he was a farmer? He didn't even finish high school, but he decided that all his kids would go to college— all seven of us. So he worked hard and did without, and took pride in each of us. He raised us to believe we could do anything." He sighs.

"That's my dad . . . And now he says he's tired, that he's ready to rest, ready to go to the Lord."

He wipes away a tear. "This is about him, now. And as much as I don't want him to go, the right thing for me to do is to honor his wishes. The right thing is to do what he wants."

"So let's try to figure out how to help your brothers and sisters understand your dad's situation and what his wishes are."

"How do we do that?"

DEVELOP A BETTER UNDERSTANDING OF THE SITUATION

I think it would be helpful if the hospice nurses and your dad's doctor communicated more regularly with your siblings. This will help them develop a more realistic view of your dad's physical condition. They have their own process to go through. If they understand how he's declining, they might choose to spend this time differently.

I'll talk with your dad and ask if we can share this information with your brothers and sisters. Even though they live outside the country, we can call them. Your doctor can, too. We can help your family find ways to cope with the situation. You don't need to do this alone.

The other thing we can do is share ideas for what they can do for him, even from far away. It's hard to feel helpless. Having something constructive to do might help everyone feel better.

LEARN WHAT'S IMPORTANT TO YOUR LOVED ONE

Your dad once shared how much he misses his home. It's unlikely he'll return. Your siblings could take a video camera to some of his favorite places. They could also record scenes of their home life, bringing loved ones together to send a greeting and news of their day.

Your siblings could tape a sunset, a sunrise, the ocean, or a mountain stream—whatever he loves and enjoys—and, with the camera on, share all the things they want to say to him, but maybe have never said. On this tape they could tell him what they learned from him, how much they admire his courage, how they carry the lessons he taught them always in their hearts, and how those lessons have helped shape their lives.

These tapes, or other things, sent regularly, either mailed or over the Internet, would be a way to share life with him, even though they're far away.

EXPLORE WHEN TO VISIT

It's likely that they'll ask you when they should visit. Truthfully, they need to make that decision for themselves. They need to decide what they want from the visit, and talk with Ferdinand about what he wants. Some people want to be there when their loved one is alert and able to have a conversation. For that I recommend that people come as soon and as often as they can. Some people want to be present near the time of death, or the time immediately following for a remembrance service. In some cultures and religious traditions, that means a lot. If people can only come once, it would be a good idea for them to examine what's most important to them, then choose.

STAY INFORMED

It's important for them to be able to talk with Ferdinand, but at a time that works for him. Rather than them calling and asking you to wake him up, they could invite your dad to call them anytime—day or night—or ask you to call for him, when he's awake and up to it. These are social calls—just to talk to him.

You'll also want to plan regularly scheduled calls to keep them informed and involved. The best way might be to get most or all your siblings on a conference call at the same time. You can do this by phone, or by using high-speed Internet you can access a free service for conference calling. By making one call with everyone on the line at once, each of your brothers and sisters gets the same information directly from you, at the same time. If you tell one of your siblings, and ask him or her to pass it on, with each retelling the story will change, even when the person relaying the information has the best of intentions.

What to Share

During the conference call consider starting the conversation by sharing your dad's reaction to the cards, letters, calls, or videos they send. Maybe share some of your own experiences, too. Like the times you and your dad laugh together, or other meaningful moments. These little details will help your siblings feel more connected, more involved in his life.

After that, provide them with a detailed, objective account of how he's doing. Remember, they don't see him as you do. Paint a picture for them of what his days preceding each call are like. Use detailed, descriptive terms. For example, tell them how many feet he's able to walk before he has to sit and rest, about how many hours per day he sleeps, the quantity and description of the foods he ate in the last twenty-four hours.

Keep notes. This way you all can see that last week he was able to walk independently twenty feet from the living room to the bathroom. This week he needs you to help him. Also, tell them about any changes in his care or medications, and what he says about how he feels. Details are important. These will help your brothers and sisters understand the changes he's undergoing. Also provide information about your dad's emotional and spiritual state. Use his actual words as often as you can recall them. This will help them better understand your dad's feelings and wishes, and help them recognize that his feelings may be different from their own.

After you've shared how he's doing, give everyone a chance to share how they feel, and, as a family, explore your values and beliefs about this process. This kind of group conversation will help each of you share your grief and work through your issues and feelings together.

Of course, make time for your Dad to participate too, if he chooses.

Changes in the Situation: Making a Plan for Communication

Another part of the communication plan would be for you to inform your siblings of any significant changes between scheduled calls. Since you likely won't have time to call all six of them, set up a system, a communication chain, where each one calls another until all are notified. The problem with that, though, is that the information will likely be reinterpreted as it's passed along. One solution might be to write the information in an e-mail, send it to everyone, then make one phone call to start the communication chain, to notify everyone to read the e-mail. There's also a free Internet service, CaringBridge, that allows you to securely post updates that your family, or others who have the password, can view.

Slowly, David nods. "I just want to do the right thing for my dad, and for my brothers and sisters. But sometimes I wonder if I'm doing enough."

I lay a gentle hand on his shoulder. "You're doing a wonderful, loving, caring job."

"He's done so much for me." He blinks back the tears that threaten to flow. "He's my dad . . ."

The most basic and powerful way to connect with another person is to listen. Just listen. Perhaps the most important thing we give each other is our attention . . . A loving silence often has more power to heal than the most well-intentioned words.

—Rachel Naomi Remen, MD

Bridging the Distance
Staying Connected

- Give your loved one a telephone calling card and invite him to call you whenever it's convenient for him.
- Video- or audiotape messages and send them frequently. Explore free or low-cost Internet resources, such as YouSendIt.com, to e-mail large digital files. See "Appendix A: Additional Resources" (page 210).
- Explore free or low-cost conference call and video communication Internet resources, such as Skype. See "Appendix A: Additional Resources" (page 210).

- Send frequent greetings via e-mail or regular mail.
- Tell your loved one, via telephone or in person, how much you value him, what you have learned from him, and the impact that learning has had on your life.

Providing Support

- Recognize the challenges faced by the caregiver. Offer the caregiver encouragement and support.
- Ask the caregiver what you can do to provide support, and determine how to provide that support.
- Explore ways to offer respite (rest) to the caregiver. Ideas include:
  Paying for a few hours of caregiving weekly.
  Organizing neighbors, friends, and church or community members to provide regular respite.
- For more suggestions, see "I Can't Do This Alone . . ." (page 71).

Managing Communication

- Establish a plan for regular communication. Consider scheduling conference calls with the primary caregiver and all significant persons. Communication should include:
  Information about what the person enjoyed since the last communication.
  Detailed, specific information about the person's physical status.
  Information about the person's emotional or spiritual feelings, using his own words, whenever possible.
  Follow up on any unresolved questions from the previous call, if still relevant.
- Allow time for each person to ask questions and share feelings.
- Establish a plan for communication between regularly scheduled calls for significant changes or urgent situations.
- Make a list of names and contact information of who should be notified about changes in his condition or other important occurrences. Keep the list updated and in an easy-to-find location.

- Consider establishing a communication chain, in which each person agrees to call the next person on the list to relay the update. The important point is for each person to continue calling until she speaks directly to someone. By simply leaving a message, a significant amount of time could pass before the information is passed on to everyone. So if the person called is not available, leave a message, then call the next person on the list, and continue calling until you speak directly to someone. Continue until the last person on the list is notified.
- Consider utilizing CaringBridge, a free Internet service to securely post updates. See "Appendix A: Additional Resources" (page 210).

Questions to Consider When Planning a Visit

- What does your loved one want?
- What do you hope for from the visit?
- Is being able to interact with your loved one important to you and your loved one?
- Is being present, or nearby, at the time of death important to you or your loved one? See "I Want to Be with Her When She Passes . . ." (page 179).
- Is attending a remembrance service important to you?
- If you are able to visit only once, what will you and your loved one value most?

I'm Exhausted!
❧ Exploring Care Settings ❧ Outside the Home
Choosing a Care Facility, If Needed, and Paying for Care

Francine and Walter

"It's just too much," Walter says, shaking his head. "If I were in better health, if our children lived closer, maybe I—" He buries his face in his hands. "I don't know what we're going to do."

I lay my arm around his shoulders, holding him until the tears subside. Finally, he lifts his head. "I should be able to do this for her," he says, wiping his eyes. "If I were stronger . . ."

"You're doing an amazing job, Walter. Taking care of a loved one is an incredibly demanding job, even for someone in good health. But the truth is, when we reach this point in life, often we're older, and our spouse is older, too. In many families, like yours, the children are grown and live far away. They're not able to take time off from their jobs to help. Oftentimes, that leaves someone like you, older, not in good health, wanting to do the best you can to take care of someone you love. This happens to a lot of people, Walter, and there are good options we can consider."

"I just want to take good care of her . . ."

"You are. And you'll still be able to take good care of her, but with help."

"How?"

"If you just need a short break, hospice can provide respite care, someone to provide the care and give you a break for up to five days, periodically. We would pay for someone to come into your home and care for her around the clock, or transfer her to another place to receive care for five days." I gauge his reaction. "But I think what you're telling me is that with your health, you'll need help continuously, beyond just a few days."

He nods and fresh tears flow. "I don't want that, but I just can't do this anymore."

"That's okay. You've done an amazing job. By finding help to take care of Francine, you'll still be there for her, you just won't be exhausted, and you won't make yourself sick. You'll be able to be with her, supporting her as her husband. And that's important."

He turns away. "We promised each other we wouldn't put the other one in some awful old folks' home. I just can't do that to her. There's got to be another way."

My arm tightens around his shoulders. "There is. There are different types of places, some are large facilities, some are family homes. Yes, some places aren't great, but there are some wonderful places, too."

"We don't have much money. Just our Social Security and a small pension. We own the house. I could sell it, I suppose, maybe move in with one of the kids. I don't really want to do that, but if I have to, to get good care for Francine . . ."

"Let's look at some options. I'll call the social worker and she'll help us figure this out."

"What do people with a lot of money do?"

"Some hire private caregivers, often through agencies, to provide care in their home, around the clock, if needed. This kind of care is usually very expensive. Some elect to move into assisted living facilities where they have their own apartment with meals, housekeeping, and some limited care services. The challenge with assisted living is that when people reach the stage where Francine is now, they'll need to move into a place that offers more complete care. Many assisted living facilities have that care on site, but it's in another building, and the rooms are arranged much like long-term-care facilities. There are also some specialized facilities that provide care to meet the unique needs of people afflicted with memory impairment, like Alzheimer's."

"So unless people can afford to hire around-the-clock help in their home, they're in the same boat I am."

I nod.

"Why doesn't Medicare cover this? All these years, I thought they did."

"A lot of people make that assumption and, like you, they're surprised, and frankly, in a difficult spot because they assume Medicare, or hospice, will provide complete care."

"If we'd understood, maybe we would have sorted all this out sooner. As it was, Francine was having to take care of me, then she got sick, and I had to try to take care of her."

"It's a good idea for people to figure this out ahead of time, when it's not a crisis. Barring a sudden death, we're all likely to need some amount of care as we age."

"It's hell getting old."

"And for all the aches and pains and challenges, I thank you for being here. One of the best parts of my job is learning from—as you call yourself—old people. With age comes a certain wisdom, a grace we just don't attain until we've seen a bit of life. Thank you."

"Well, you're welcome, I think." He chuckles, then turns serious. "If Francine goes somewhere else, will we still get hospice care?"

"Yes. There's one exception, called a skilled nursing facility. Skilled nursing care includes things like rehabilitation. Medicare won't cover this kind of care and hospice at the same time. But we're not talking about that kind of care for Francine, so that's not an issue."

"Good. I'm glad we'll still have hospice to help us."

"Let's look at some options. First, let's talk about what resources might be available to help pay for the care, then let's explore what kind of care setting is right for you and Francine."

PAYING FOR CARE

It's possible that you and Francine might qualify for Supplemental Security Income, a federal benefit. It's also possible you might qualify for Medicaid. The qualification rules for Medicaid vary by state, and whether the person needing assistance is married or single. For married couples, Medicaid recognizes that the other partner will still need a place to live and funds to live on, so, in most states, Medicaid allows married couples to keep their house. To see if you meet the financial qualifications, they'll look at your income and any assets you have besides your home, furnishings, and personal items. They'll also look at Francine's care needs. If she needed care for only a few hours a day, it's likely they'd pay to have someone come to your home. But since she needs care around the clock, she'll probably need to go somewhere else, to some kind of group setting. You'll have a number of choices available, and it will be up to you and Francine to choose the right one.

I'll ask the social worker to meet with you and start looking into whether you qualify for these and other federal, state, and local benefit programs. If you, or your kids, want to do some checking, you can research this on the Internet.

Costs for care can vary widely, depending on amenities and services, but in most communities, you'll find both large facilities and private foster homes that accept Medicaid, or offer care at the lower end of the price scale.

OPTIONS FOR CARE

Let's start with an option you may not be familiar with—adult foster homes. Most people have never heard of adult foster homes. They're private homes of families who choose to take in people, like Francine, who need basic care. You don't really notice them. They're tucked into neighborhoods, just like all the other homes. The homeowners mow their lawn; their kids ride bikes in the street; and the only thing different about them is that there are often a few older folks, some in wheelchairs, sitting out on the front porch, enjoying the day.

Adult foster homes are licensed and regularly inspected to ensure that they maintain good standards of care. In most places, residents have their own room and can also spend time in living areas with the family and other residents. Adult foster homes provide care for only a few residents at a time, and they're able to take care of people over the entire course of their illness, right up to the end. So if you do choose an adult foster home, Francine won't have to move as her needs change.

Many of these places are operated by people from other cultures. I meet a lot of foster home providers from Eastern Europe and Southeast Asia. In their cultures, older people are honored, more so, perhaps, than in our culture.

Adult foster homes can be wonderful places that provide great care. You can also consider a large facility, what we commonly think of as a nursing home. There are some really good facilities that provide excellent care.

Choosing the Right Care Provider

The social worker can give you a list of adult foster homes and nursing facilities that have a vacancy and accept the type of payment—be it Medicaid or something else—that you and the social worker determine is available. You, or you and your family, will need to choose the place. It's up to you to decide what you and Francine are comfortable with.

You'll probably want to call first and ask some questions. Of those that sound like they might be a good fit, check the state's department of health and human services for complaints. The social worker can help with that.

Next, arrange a visit. You might consider asking one of your children to fly in and help you choose. In the meantime, we can arrange for respite, for Francine to be cared for, for up to five days, to give you time to look.

Plan to spend some time in the places you're considering. Walk around. Talk to the residents and other families. Do the residents look happy? Do the staff or family providing care look happy? Are the residents out in the common areas or gardens? Does the food look good? Do the facilities look clean? Does it smell clean? Does the place feel peaceful?

You'll also want to consider how close it is to your home. How easy will it be for you to visit? What are the visiting hours? Will you have a peaceful setting where you can visit? Will you have privacy where you can talk?

Ask if the routine can be adapted as Francine's needs change. For example, when she's no longer able to eat a full meal at mealtime, will they offer her snacks? When she's close to passing, will you be able to be with her, no matter what time of day or night? Is there a comfortable chair or cot available for you to sleep beside her?

If you're considering an adult foster home run by people from another culture, ask if there is always someone in the home who speaks English. You'll also want to ask what kind of food they prepare. Most places, even those run by people of other cultures, prepare the kind of foods Francine is used to, but it's good to ask.

What it really comes down to, Walter, is this: Do you feel comfortable there? Will Francine? It won't be home, but does it feel like a good place to be? I think, Walter, you'll know it when you find it.

Most important, you need to know that you haven't failed Francine in any way. A lot of families face this same challenge. Despite everyone's best effort, they're just not able to provide care in the home. But there are good places for care besides your home. The silver lining is that with others providing the physical care, you'll have more time and energy to be with Francine as a husband, and not an exhausted caregiver. You'll be able to just be with her, hold her hand, talk with her, sit with her while she sleeps, whatever feels right for you.

"That would be really nice," Walter says. He reaches for my hand. "I don't feel so wise right now, just old. Old, and a little scared."

"I read this once, years ago: 'Life is not a journey to the grave with the intention of arriving safely in a pretty and well-preserved body, but rather to skid in broadside, thoroughly used up, totally worn out, and loudly proclaiming, Wow, What a ride!' "

He chuckles. "Well, that would be Francine and me . . . What a ride."

Epilogue

With the help of a social worker, Walter found a good adult foster home near their home. Francine had her own room. From her window they could watch the family's children play in the yard. Walter spent most of each day with her, in a comfortable recliner beside her bed. As her time grew short, he was able to spend the night at her side, and was with her when she died.

I do not understand the mystery of grace—only that it meets us where we are, but does not leave us where it found us.

—Anne Lamott

HIRING ADDITIONAL CAREGIVING HELP

Questions for Discussion

- What are the goals for care? Goals might include:
  Ensuring comfort.
  Meeting basic needs (toileting, bathing, repositioning, etc.).
  Ensuring that the caregiver is physically able to provide care.
  Ensuring that caregiver(s) aren't overwhelmed.
  Establishing a sense of calm and peacefulness.
  Providing everyone with an opportunity to find meaning and closure.
- Are you able to meet these goals at home?
- What are the obstacles to meeting these goals?
- What resources might be available to overcome these obstacles? For support ideas, see "I Can't Do This Alone . . ." (page 71).
- If obstacles can't be overcome, is care in another setting a way to meet the goals?
- What financial resources are available to pay for care? For more information, see "Appendix A: Additional Resources" (page 210).
- After exploring these issues, do you feel that the decision you've reached best meets everyone's needs?
- Can you accept this decision and go forward with a sense of peace and greater ability to enjoy the time remaining?

Caregiving Options
In-Home Caregivers

For round-the-clock care, in-home, paid caregiving is one of the most expensive options. In most midsized and larger communities, staffing agencies can arrange care for a fee. The agency is responsible for screening, hiring, scheduling, and paying wages, taxes, and benefits for qualified caregivers. You will be charged an hourly rate that includes the caregivers' wages and an agency fee. Most professional home caregiving is performed by nurse's aides. Rates vary by community. For more information, see "Appendix A: Additional Resources" (page 210).

Alternative Care Settings
Short-Term Alternatives

Respite Care: Provides up to five days of care, either in your home or in a long-term care facility (offered and paid for by Medicare-licensed hospice providers).

Inpatient Hospital Care: Utilized when a person's symptoms, such as pain, delirium, shortness of breath, or other distressing symptoms, cannot be managed in the current setting, whether at home or in a care facility. The person is temporarily hospitalized for treatment. Once stabilized, the person will be discharged. Hospitalization may also be called for when death is imminent (twenty-four to forty-eight hours) if the family or caregivers feel they are unable to cope with the event in the current setting. This option is offered and paid for by Medicare-licensed hospice providers.

Longer-Term Alternatives

Assisted Living Facility: Provides a range of supportive care that varies by facility and state. Talk with your local hospice to learn more about the level of care provided by ALFs in your community. When selecting an ALF, choose a facility that can meet your needs now and in the future. Ask if total care is available and where that care is provided. In some ALFs, total care can be provided within the resident's apartment. In others, the resident will need to move to a different location within the complex or off-site. Not all ALFs provide this level of care.

Long-Term Care/Nursing Home: Provides twenty-four-hour supportive care; the majority of care is provided by nurse's aides, with RN's on site. Facilities are often large, with semiprivate rooms, and are able to meet increasing care needs throughout the process. Staff changes two to three times in a twenty-four-hour period.

Adult Foster Care Home: Provides twenty-four-hour supportive care in a home setting. Care is provided by trained family and staff who meet state standards. Like all care facilities, adult foster homes are regulated, licensed, and inspected by the state. Rooms are generally private. The number of residents receiving care is often small. Adult foster homes are able to provide care throughout the process.

Skilled Nursing Care: Provides twenty-four-hour supportive care plus skilled care, which may include regular physical therapy, extensive dressing changes, or intravenous medication management. This care is paid for by Medicare or other insurance. To qualify for this level of care, a person must have been hospitalized for at least three days, and have a need for skilled care, such as rehabilitation, which is ordered by a physician. Be aware that Medicare hospice cannot be provided with this level of care.

Choosing among Professional Caregiving Options

- Obtain the assistance of a social worker through hospice, the hospital, or your county's Office of Aging Services.
- Determine your available financial resources. See "Appendix A: Additional Resources" (page 210). If you purchased long-term-care insurance, review your policy and contact the insurance carrier.
- Explore and discuss your feelings about hiring in-home care or moving your loved one to a care facility. See Questions for Discussion above.
- Develop criteria, including:
  Proximity

Type of setting (adult foster home, large care facility, etc.)

Form of payment accepted

+ With the assistance of the social worker, determine whether there are openings in facilities that meet your criteria.

+ Check references. Check state records for complaints.

+ Visit the best matches. Evaluate:

Quality of care

Flexibility of care

Caregivers' interactions with residents and their families

Overall Environment

After Placement in a Care Facility or Hiring In-home Care

+ Remain informed and continue to participate in care decisions.

+ Ask questions as needed.

+ Visit frequently to ease the transition for all.

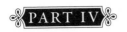

PART IV

Closure: Will I Die a "Good" Death?

This section offers information that may be of value to individuals seeking meaning as their life nears its end, and to family members supporting a loved one through this process. Not all chapters will be relevant to your situation, so read only what you feel applies to you.

In this section you'll explore some of the challenges people may face as they review their life and search for meaning. You'll discover how others have addressed these issues, and how they resolved them. You'll find practical tips as well as discussion questions to help you explore your own feelings to achieve resolution, meaning, and peace.

I'm Afraid to Lose Control . . .
Examining the Fear of Loss of Control and Discovering Ways to Achieve Peace

I'm Not Ready . . .
Making the Most of the Time You Have

Is It Too Late to Make Amends?
Achieving Reconciliation, Forgiveness, and Healing

I'm Ready—Why Am I Not Going?
Understanding and Achieving Acceptance and Peace

Why Me? Why Am I Being Punished?
Reconciling Mortality with Your Religious Beliefs

We Always Thought We'd Have More Time . . .
Realizing Dreams and Appreciating the Choices You Have Made

I'M AFRAID TO
✿ LOSE CONTROL... ✿

*Examining the Fear of Loss of Control and
Discovering Ways to Achieve Peace*

Helen

"I'VE BEEN IN CHARGE ALL MY LIFE. I can't stomach the idea of becoming dependent on someone, having to ask for everything," says Helen. Now in her late sixties, she has worked as a model since her teens. But a cancer diagnosis eight months ago and the resulting disfigurement changed all that, robbing her of her livelihood and much of her self-image. Its continued advance now threatens to rob her of her independence, which is central to her life.

"I grew up with a mother who always had to scrape through life on what my father would or wouldn't allow. He made her feel like she was nothing—that he was everything. I told myself that wasn't for me. So I got out of there as soon as I could. I made my own way. Nobody was going to tell me what to do.

"And now the doctors are telling me that I can't beat this cancer. That I'll get weaker, that I'll need my daughter, or someone else to take care of me." She shakes her head. "I've fought all my life. I'm not going to stop fighting now."

"What are you fighting?" I ask.

"I can't beat the cancer. I accept that. But I can decide how I'm going to die. I'm going to be in control of this, right up to the end."

"So being in control is important to you."

"Damn right."

"I suspect that right now you don't feel completely in control, and that's really difficult for you."

"I've been told I'm going to die. How does that leave me with any control?"

"Is it that you feel you're not in control, or that you feel you don't have choices?"

"What?"

"You've gone through life deciding what you want, then going after it. I suspect that, for the most part, by working hard you've managed to get what you want. Perhaps for you, control is being able to make things happen the way you want them to. But try as you might, you can't bring about a recovery. You can't achieve the outcome you want. So now you push back, with anger, and I can't blame you. But you do have choices."

Her composure fails. Tears begin to stream down her face. "What choice could I possibly have right now?"

"Right now, you're angry. And that's okay. As bad as anger feels, it's part of the process, and it's healthy to express it, to let it out. The choice you have, though, is this: Do you continue to be angry, or do you find a way to see beyond the anger and find something else?

"Some people never get past it. No matter what they do, they can't attain what they want, and they just get stuck in that frustration, that anger.

"Some, though, are able to come to terms with the situation. Yes, there is a time to fight, but in our fighting, do we lose what we're fighting for? If we're fighting to live, what is living?"

"What do you mean?"

"While trying to hold on to what we're afraid we'll lose, do we lose the ability to enjoy it? This is the choice we all face, no matter how long our life may be. Every one of us dies. Most of us just don't know when.

"Every day we have a choice about how we live. Do we go through life grasping for every little thing, struggling to hold on to things we're afraid to lose, or do we live open to what may come? Yes, life brings losses, but it also brings good things. Are we able to open ourselves, or are we so closed around what we have that the rest just passes us by?"

"What good things? What good comes from dying?"

"Peace. Closure. Resolution. Understanding . . ."

"And you think I can find peace?" she says, part rebuttal, part question.

"Do you want to?"

Her turquoise eyes widen.

"In that, too, you have a choice. We don't control what happens to us, but we do control how we respond to it. If you want to find peace, I believe you'll find it."

She stares at me, then whispers, "How?"

"What is peace to you?"

After a long pause, she answers. "Peace would be not having to fight."

"Then don't fight. Just live. Today. Tomorrow. Whatever comes. Yes, it's likely you'll lose your independence, that you'll need your daughter to help you. Look at it as a gift of being able to spend this time with her.

"Every night when you fall asleep, think about the good things that happened that day, seeing your daughter smile, a bird singing outside your window, the memory of a good friend. Yes, you will have losses, but you choose what you think about. And what you think about, in many ways, becomes who you are."

"Do you believe that?" she asks.

"Yes. I also believe it's not easy to change habits developed over a lifetime, habits attached to how we think, how we react. As hard as this end-of-life journey can be, I think it teaches us the richest lessons life offers. It's too bad we often wait until the end to learn them.

"Some people, though, never do. For them, what they perceive as loss of control is too much, so they opt to end it early, or they remain mired in their frustration and anger and die quite badly. But there, too, lies a choice."

"By 'end it early' you mean suicide." She turns toward the window. "What do you tell people who come to you and ask for help to end it?" Her gaze remains on the trees outside her window.

"I don't tell them anything. I listen. If they're considering it, they have strong reasons for doing so. The best way I can help is to understand what they fear, what they want to avoid, what has led them to consider this choice."

For a long time she says nothing. Finally, she asks, "And once you know why, what do you do?"

"Sometimes what leads people to this point is fear of the unknown. 'What will happen? How will it happen? How will I deal with it?' At times, that fear can be overwhelming. If they fear pain or other symptoms, we help them understand how we will keep them comfortable. But for a lot of people, fear of pain or other symptoms is only part of the reason."

She takes a deep breath. "I think you know what I'm afraid of."

I wait.

"I'm afraid to lose control," she says at last.

"You have control. You control how you respond to what happens in life. You choose, every step of the way. And yes, you can choose to end it—but you can also choose how you live. Yes, your body will decline; it will fail. But you are more than your body. Far more."

She considers my words, then says, "I'm afraid of something else."

I wait.

"You said some people die badly. What does that mean? Can you change that, too?"

"It's something you change. That, too, is part of your choice. In all the years I've been doing this, I've learned that we die much the way we have lived. If we've been open, generous, and kind in our living, it's likely we'll make this final passage with that same calm grace. If we've spent our lives struggling for control, always fearful, always holding tight to what we have, then in death we'll also struggle—against the loss of control, against the unknown, against letting go. But even then, in our final months, weeks, days even, we have a choice.

"Some people can become so overwhelmed by their need for control that they lose the ability to cope. Watching them, it's like watching someone try to fight his way out, except there's nothing tangible to fight. They become restless, agitated, even combative with their loved ones.

"We can offer sedation, if the family chooses, but even then, watching these people, I still wonder how much of that struggle continues within."

"How so?"

"I remember one man. He'd struggled to control everything all his life. When things didn't go his way, he'd resort to abuse—verbal and physical. He was that way with everyone—his coworkers, strangers in a bar, even his wife and children.

"Everyone tried to help him cope, but he just became more agitated. One night, when he could barely rise from a chair, he summoned every bit of strength he had and tried to run. When his legs failed and we tried to help him, he just started swinging—at us, at his family, at thin air.

"For the next few days he had this wild look of an enraged, terrified animal. No one could get close without him becoming violent. Finally, his family decided to sedate him, thinking that might give him peace.

"He'd lie in bed, no longer fighting, no longer able to respond. His eyes were open, but even with all that medication, he never lost that frightened, animal-like look. The skin on his face was taut, as if he were gritting his teeth. He lived like this longer than any of us thought possible.

"One day as I stood beside his bed, the heavy gray clouds that had filled the sky broke, and the sun emerged. Light flooded the room and bathed his face with this warm, golden hue. I remember watching his face in this light, watching as the muscles relaxed, as the look in his eyes calmed. He drew a deep breath. Then another. And another. And a few moments later, he was gone.

"I stood beside him for a moment, wondering what had happened, what brought about the changes I saw. Did he finally find release, forgiveness, acceptance, redemption? Or was the light merely a coincidence, and the change in his face an illusion?"

"What do you think it was?"

"I don't know. Whatever it was, whatever happened in his final moments, I hope he found peace."

"I'd rather not end up like that." For a long time she gazes out the window. Then she turns to me. "Do I really have a choice?"

"Yes. I believe you do. I believe it because I see it happen all the time. You really can choose how you make this journey." Then, in a quiet voice, I ask, "What will you choose?"

Again, she turns to the window. Finally, she answers. "I've spent all my life working: to look the way I do, to choose the right people to have around me, to build my career. And I always wanted options. No matter what choice I made, I always wanted to know I had a way out." She pauses. "And there's a way out of this, too."

I wait.

"But maybe, for once, that's not the point," she says. "Maybe, for all this, for all the things I've been thinking I'll lose, maybe there's something . . ." Then, with a stronger voice, she continues. "Maybe this is the lesson you were talking about. We go through life so busy planning, so busy struggling to always be in control that we miss out on what happens . . . or can happen, if we only let it.

"Maybe, for once in my life, I don't have to be in control. I just get to enjoy. My daughter's smile. The autumn sunshine. Rain on the falling leaves. Winter . . . Maybe I'll live to see spring. But if I don't . . . Maybe just enjoying today is enough." She closes her eyes. "Maybe that's peace."

God, grant me the serenity to accept the things I cannot change, the courage to change the things I can, and the wisdom to know the difference.
—Reinhold Niebuhr

DEVELOPING A "WISH LIST"

Consider developing a list of what you hope to do or experience in the time that remains, as well as a description of how you'd like to spend your final days or hours. "To Do or Experience" items might include spending time with loved ones, writing letters to close friends, giving away treasured possessions, or mending strained relationships. For more ideas, see "We Always Thought We Had More Time" (page 152), and the sidebar, "Suggestions for Achieving Closure" (page 136).

In exploring how you wish to spend your final days or hours, consider that it's likely you will be only minimally conscious of what's happening around you. You may be able to hear, but not able to interact in any other way. You may also be conscious of other things and may wish to be more engaged with these experiences. (See "Will I Be Alone?" page 6.) As you express your wishes for your final days or hours, recognize that your feelings about how you spend this time and what you want to happen around you may change as you experience this passage.

Questions to Consider

- Do you want to be at home? If so, in what room?
- Do you want to be near a window?
- Who would you like near you?
- Given that you may be able to hear, would you like some form of sound at low volume? Ideas might include: gently flowing water, soft music, the reading of scriptures, some other sound, or silence.
- What would you like in the room? Ideas might include photos of loved ones, religious objects, or other items of special meaning to you.

Loved ones and caregivers attempting to honor these requests must realize that circumstances may not allow for every request to be honored exactly as the person specified. Honor these requests as best you can, recognizing that situations change, and that no one can truly anticipate what she will experience or want until this time arrives. For more information about creating a peaceful environment and expressing wishes for the final days or hours, see "I Want to Be with Her When She Passes . . ." (page 179).

❋ I'm Not Ready... ❋
Making the Most of the Time You Have

Christopher and Paige

"GOOD LUCK!" WE WISH CHRISTOPHER as he wheels past the nurses' station, en route to his oncologist. Christopher grins and waves, but his wife, Paige, stares straight ahead, frowning as she pushes the wheelchair down the hall. For the past seven years they have fought Christopher's cancer. For seven years, this disease—this battle—has defined their family's life.

Christopher came to the hospice house a week before, suffering from severe nausea and plummeting blood counts. His oncologist called a halt to chemotherapy. When Christopher insisted that he could continue, the oncologist was adamant: "You won't survive it."

Our task was to gain control over the nausea and stabilize him. And now, nausea free, his blood counts restored, Christopher wants to resume the chemo. "Come to the office. We'll evaluate you, but I make no promises," the oncologist warns.

Four hours later, Christopher and Paige return to the hospice, their faces grim. I draw up a syringe of medication and without a word, follow them down the hall.

"I can't do this anymore!" Paige snaps as they cross the threshold of Christopher's room.

"We can't give up," Christopher pleads. "I'm not ready to die!"

"Damn it. It's always about you!"

I close their door and wait outside, wondering what it would be like to be in their place, raising two teenage daughters, keeping a marriage together, fighting this all-consuming battle with cancer. Finally, the door swings open and Paige storms past. Christopher turns toward the window and stares at the woods beyond.

"I brought some medication," I say. Christopher lifts his arm and I infuse the medicine in his IV. Then I check the other IV lines, the tubes, the pumps, the drains, the dressings. Everything is as it should be, despite the car ride, the hours at the hospital, the tests, the disappointment. I turn to leave.

"The tumors have grown," Christopher says. "Will you sit with me? Just for a little while?"

I settle on the window seat, near his wheelchair. For a long time, neither of us says a word.

He is at his best when his daughters, Chelsea and Annie, visit. Young, pretty, and poised, the girls have known little else beyond the daily round of hospitals and doctors and medicines. For nearly half their lives, their dad has been sick. For a brief period when Chelsea, the eldest, was twelve, it looked as if Christopher would beat the disease, and for two years this family attempted to create a normal life with soccer games, family vacations, and dance recitals. But the cancer returned, and once again cancer rules their lives.

When the girls visit, Christopher's face lights up and his boyish laughter joyfully flows. He helps with homework and draws from each daughter stories about her day. In listening to these evening visits, one can imagine this scene taking place in a home, not a hospice.

But this is a hospice, and while Christopher revels in his evenings with his daughters, he avoids his wife, she avoids him, and everyone avoids the truth.

"I wish she were different," he says.

"This disease has taken its toll on everyone."

"I didn't ask for this. If I could give them a normal life . . . I want that more than anything." He turns away. Then he sighs. "It's as if she resents that I'm sick, that we can't do the things normal families do, that the girls spend their evenings at a hospital, or home with me, instead of out with their friends. It's as if I'm standing in the way of everything she wants for them. Honestly, I think she'd be happier if I didn't make it."

"Have you talked with her about this?"

He shakes his head. "When? She's never here. Now that Chelsea drives, Paige doesn't need to bring the girls to see me." He plucks at the blanket that covers his legs. "Maybe when we get past this one . . . When I'm home again, maybe things will get better."

I glance at the tubes and pumps, the array of technology that keeps him alive. "What has your doctor told you?"

"He says I won't beat this." He lifts his chin. "Do you know how many times I've heard that?"

"But what if you don't?"

Christopher's eyes widen, and I continue. "Have you talked with your wife about what you both want for your children, and how you can make that happen? Have you talked with her about how to use this time to help the girls, after you're gone?"

He doesn't answer. Finally, he says, "I have to stay alive. I have to . . . for them." His voice breaks. "I know I can't beat this, but if I can just stay alive long enough to be there . . . to help them grow up. I'm not ready to go. I can't give up hope."

"I know you hope for more time, but do you hope for other things as well? Like the kind of future you want for your children, and how you want them to remember you, the lessons you want to leave them with?

"How you live has taught them about joy and love, determination and courage. But what else do you want for them as they grow up, as they live their lives, as they, someday, raise their own children? Perhaps that, too, is something to hope for."

"I can't think about that. I just have to keep fighting."

And this remains the driving motivation in Christopher's life. Every choice he makes, he makes to buy time. The cancer continues to spread. But he fights on, cherishing his evenings with his girls, never speaking of his illness, never seeing, never speaking to his wife.

One evening the fight ends. But it does not end well. Instead of a peaceful journey, with all the words said, the advice, the hopes, the dreams communicated, the problems addressed, the future for his children more certain, he dies with nothing resolved. He leaves a void that could, perhaps, have been filled. He leaves a family with a hole. He is gone. But he never said good-bye.

Jewell and Her Family

Jewell comes to us for many of the same reasons but, in the end, she makes a different choice than Christopher did. She, too, lives tethered to machines, with tubes poking in and out of her body. She chooses this life because it brings one more day with her nine-year-old daughter, Annabel. Every day the cancer advances, and every day she makes the choice to continue to fight—one more surgery, one more machine. Her mother, Evelyn, tells her she must fight at all costs. Her husband Oliver merely sits quietly at her bedside and holds her hand. When Jewell asks him what he thinks she should do, he replies that she alone should decide.

One afternoon the argument in Jewell's room is especially loud as Evelyn hammers home her point. "If you just lie there, you're not going to get better! Your husband is incapable of making decisions for you, and as tired as you are all the time, it's too much for you to fight the doctors for what you need. Let me make the decisions. We're not ready to give up. You've got to keep fighting.

"Listen to me," Evelyn snaps. "I have to do this for you. I have to take care of you. And I have to take care of Annabel. What if the worst happens and you don't make it? Annabel needs someone strong. I'll get a lawyer to draw up the papers. I'll make decisions for you, and if—*if*—you don't make it, then I'll raise Annabel."

I step into the room and Evelyn glares at me. "What do you want?"

"I need to change Jewell's dressings. Would you mind stepping outside for a few minutes?" In truth, the dressings could be changed later. But changing them now might give Jewell a little breathing room to collect her thoughts, to decide what she wants to do, to prepare an answer for her mother.

Evelyn steps out and I close the door. As I arrange supplies, I ask Jewell, "Have you talked with her about what *you* want?"

She shakes her head. I sit beside the bed.

"My doctor said he'd never give up, but he gave up," she says, expelling a shaking breath. "He said there are no more options, no more treatments." She pauses. "My mother says I should keep fighting, but my doctor says nothing more can be done to try to cure me or keep me alive any longer." She reaches for a tissue and wipes her eyes.

"What do you think?" I ask. "Do you think anything more can be done to extend your life?"

She stares at the tissue wadded in her hand. "There's not much left of me . . . What am I going to do? What would you do?"

This is her journey, and that answer—what is right for her—must come from her. But I can offer a place to start, to help her sort things out so she can make her choice. "I think I would try to find some quiet time alone," I offer. "I think I would ask myself, 'If I only have a few weeks left, how do I want to spend them? What memories do I want to make for those I'll leave behind? What can I do to touch the lives of those I love, to let them know that I love them? How do I want to say good-bye?'

"Some people, especially those with younger children, write letters to be opened in the years to come. Some make video or audio recordings. Some like to spend quiet time just being together. Whatever you decide, we can help."

Jewell turns away. "I'd like to be alone now. Can you change the dressings later?"

That day Jewell makes her choice. She will not live to see her daughter grow up, but she can be there in spirit. She banishes all argument from her room, making it clear to her mother and her husband that the life she dreams of for her daughter does not include conflict between them, and that they must work together to raise Annabel, with love and respect.

In the evenings after Annabel leaves, Jewell closes her eyes and imagines a moment she will not live to see. Then she picks up a pen and begins to write a series of letters.

My Dearest Annabel . . . For your 13th birthday . . . As you graduate . . . As you follow your dreams to sing and dance . . . For your wedding day . . . For the day when you, too, become a mother . . .

Epilogue

Recently, the local newspaper printed an article about a poised young lady who realized her dream to sing the lead role in a musical theater production. Years ago the girl's mother had passed away after a long battle with cancer. As the audience applauded, the girl stepped forward and took a bow. Her father, beaming, placed in her arms a bouquet of long-stemmed red roses, and a letter from her mom.

Courage is the price life extracts for granting peace.

—Amelia Earhart

SUGGESTIONS FOR ACHIEVING CLOSURE

- Be selective in using your energy. Choose the people with whom you wish to spend time.

- Don't wait to have meaningful conversations. Ask yourself: If I never have another chance to talk with someone I care about, what do I want her to know? Your remaining time together will likely be more meaningful having shared these feelings.

- Look for ways to realize your dreams now. See "We Always Thought We'd Have More Time . . ." (page 152).

- Consider writing letters, or making audio or video recordings for future occasions.

- Give treasured possessions to those you love now. Savor the joy they feel in receiving these special mementos from you.

- Resolve open issues. Say, "I love you," or "I'm sorry," or "I forgive you."

- Forgive yourself.

Is It Too Late to Make Amends?

Achieving Reconciliation, Forgiveness, and Healing

Rebecca

Estranged from her family, Rebecca sits with our chaplain, and anyone else who will listen, and chews on the events of her life—the choices she has made, the people she has hurt, what she has lost, and the values she held that she now realizes were unimportant.

"Why am I still alive?" she asks. "There must be a reason—something I still have to do." Day after day she shares her regrets, clinging to her burdens, for without them, what would she be? Her identity, her former sense of self, she has now rejected. Her identity now centers on remorse.

One day, as she repeats the litany of the losses she feels because of all that she didn't understand, I interrupt and ask, "What about now?"

She flinches. "What?"

"What about now? Can you change what you do because of what you now understand?"

She turns away, stammering. I reach for her hand and hold it, though perhaps she would rather pull away. "Can you let go of the past? Can you live now? Can you take that understanding of what you have done, what you haven't done in your life, and use it to now be the person you want to be?"

"There's no time."

I smile. "There's right now. There's today. What are you going to do with today? If this is your very last day, what are you going to do with it?"

She stares at me. Then she asks, "Do you think today is my last day?"

"No. I think we're stuck with you a while longer."

Seeing my grin, she breaks into a deep laugh. "Glad to know I have at least *some* use!" As our laughter subsides, she turns serious and asks, "What do you think I should do?"

I shrug. "I don't know. It's your life. Maybe ask yourself, 'What's most important to me?' Maybe start there."

"I don't know if my kids even want to talk to me."

"Do you want to talk to them?"

She nods. "Yes, I do."

"What do you want them to know?"

She sits quietly for a moment, then answers. "A lot of things. Starting with the fact that I'm sorry. I'm sorry it's taken me so long to figure this out. I still haven't got it right, but at least I see things more clearly now." She sighs. "There's so much . . . so much to say, so much time I've lost . . . And what you're telling me, I think, is that I can lose this time, too, or I can do something . . . something good with it."

"It's up to you."

Lizzy and Her Family

For some families, the time to sit together, to ask forgiveness, to be forgiven, appears lost as their loved one hovers near death, unable to speak, unable to respond in any way. Yet, even then, the chance to reconcile still exists.

One afternoon a family of siblings gathers. Word has spread that Lizzy, the youngest, lies unresponsive, hours away from death. In the small room, the tension is palpable as the factions of siblings choose their space, maintaining an unspoken agreement to interact with bare civility. "We haven't spoken in a long time," Richard, the eldest brother, confides.

"But you've come together now," I say.

"Not exactly . . . But she's our sister. We've all had our differences with her, and with each other, but we couldn't let her die alone."

Late in the afternoon, one sister takes her place beside the bed. She takes Lizzy's hand and begins to sob. "I'm sorry. I'm so sorry I wasn't the sister I could have been. I should have been there for you. All these years . . . I'm so sorry." She waits, tears flowing, hoping for some kind of response. But Lizzy is beyond that now.

Still, the sister continues, recalling and sobbing. I watch, listening as the list of hurts and misunderstandings mounts, feeling helpless to relieve this horrible suffering. Then I lay a gentle hand on the crying woman's arm. "You cannot change the past. It's gone. All you have is *this* moment."

The woman stares up at me. Then the pain in her face changes to a soft light. She draws Lizzy's hand to her cheek. She remains at the bedside, gently stroking Lizzy until she passes in this quiet space two hours later.

I often wonder, later, in the days and years that followed: Did this woman reach beyond the past for her other sisters' hands, for her brothers' hands? Did she try to make amends, or at least try to start anew? Did losing Lizzy, with so many wounds unhealed, lead her to try to heal other wounds with her other brothers and sisters, within herself?

The world is three days: As for yesterday, it has vanished, along with all that was in it. As for tomorrow, you may never see it. As for today, it is yours, so work on it.

—Hassan al-Basri

Suggestions for Achieving Reconciliation

- What are you asking forgiveness for?
- From whom are you asking forgiveness?
- Going forward, can you change the behaviors for which you are apologizing? To ask forgiveness then continue the behaviors for which you seek forgiveness holds no meaning.
- If you are seeking reconciliation of past, broken relationships, explore your motives.
- Will you feel resolution if you apologize, or only if the person accepts your apology?

- Does your happiness depend on how someone responds, or only on yourself? Remember, you cannot control what others do. You are responsible only for your own actions and your own responses to the actions of others.
- Consider involving an intermediary to convey your desire for peace and forgiveness.
- If the person you seek forgiveness from is receptive to a meeting, arrange one as soon as possible. At the meeting, be prepared to listen as well as speak.
- If the person you seek forgiveness from is not willing to meet, consider writing a letter or making an audio- or videotape expressing what you want to say, perhaps stating your apology, and reflecting on the lessons you've learned and how you'll apply these lessons to shape your remaining life. Ask an intermediary to convey to the person with whom you would like to make amends that you have written a letter or made a tape. Perhaps someday the person will be willing to read or hear your words.
- Accept the outcome, whether good or bad. Hold to the grace you found to face and accept responsibility for your mistakes.
- Let go of the past. Forgive yourself.
- Go forward, free of the burden of guilt and remorse.
- Live now. In your spirit and your actions, be the person you want to be.

I'm Ready—
Why Am I Not Going?

Understanding and Achieving Acceptance and Peace

Stan

"I'm ready to go. I wait, but nothing happens," Stan says as we sit together in his room at the assisted living facility. "I've done everything I need to do, taken care of everything. Why am I still here? I'm tired of living . . . I'm tired of living here. The food is bad. The bed is uncomfortable. I can't get a decent night's sleep without somebody waking me up to check on me. I don't have any friends. The only person who comes to see me is my nephew, and he only comes because he thinks I'll leave him all my money. I can't stand him." Stan turns to me. "Do you like me?"

I smile. For some reason I really do like this grouchy, miserly man. When I tell him this, he shakes his head. "But I have nothing to give you. Why would you like me?"

"Do you think people like one another simply because of what they can get?"

He nods, then leans close, his voice dropping to a whisper. "You should see the women here. In their eighties, chasing after me like I was Don Juan. Making me cookies, inviting me to coffee . . . The other day, one lady even put her hand on my leg. Broad daylight. In the dining room." He wags a finger at me. "It's because I have money. Plain and simple. They don't give a hoot about me. It's my money they're after."

"So let me see if I've got this straight," I say. "You've got all these women chasing after you, yet all you do is complain. You say you don't have friends, but what about these ladies? Do you think they might want something so simple, so enriching as friendship? They're widows. They're alone, just like you."

Stan frowns. "How do I know they're not out to steal me blind?"

He shakes his head. "I just want to get this over with. Why am I not going?"

So far, nothing I or any of the other team members have offered Stan has made any difference in his outlook on life. So I decide to tell him about Ishi.

"Who's Ishi?" he asks. "And what kind of name is that?"

"Japanese."

"Oh." He frowns.

I continue anyway. "Ishi was about as different from you as a person can get."

"Then why are you telling me this?"

"Because you asked me a question. Because you've been asking me and everyone else on the team the same question for weeks now. You're frustrated and unhappy. So I'm going to tell you about Ishi."

"Okay, okay. Tell me about Ishi. Though I doubt it will do any good."

"Probably not."

He frowns, then begins to laugh. "I'm not an easy man to be around." He pats my hand. "Was Ishi? Was he easy to be around?"

"He was a very kind, gentle man. He always smiled."

"And I always frown."

"But you can work on that."

"Get on with your story."

"Ah yes, Ishi . . . Like you, he said the same thing: 'I'm ready to go.' But unlike you, his was a very happy, peaceful journey. He said good-bye to his family, and with a smile on his face and openness in his heart, passed away soon after."

"How'd he do that?"

I hesitate, searching for words: How to explain to Stan the difference between choosing to let go and actually letting go? "I think, Stan, for you, letting go is about leaving this life behind. Frankly, an unhappy life. You're done with this. You find no pleasure. You want to just close your eyes and be done with it.

"But I don't think it works like that. Not that anyone really knows. All I can share with you is what I've seen. And it seems to me that the people who make the choice to let go and then linger, quite unhappily, are a lot like you. They're unhappy about their past and not happy with what's happening now. Or there are other people who are so anxious to get to what's next—whatever that is for them—that they completely lose sight of being here now. They say to me, 'I'm ready to join the Lord. Why isn't he taking me, now?'

"I think, Stan, the people who make the choice to let go, then really do let go and pass peacefully soon after, have a completely different view about life, about living, about what it means to let go. They come from many different backgrounds, different cultures, have different spiritual beliefs. Yet the one thing they seem to have in common is a sense of peace, of acceptance. It's as if they've been able to let go of the past and accept it for what it is. They no longer feel the need or responsibility to control what happens, now or in the future. They're able to live this moment, without judgment, or recrimination, or worry. And if they believe in a higher being, they seem to hold the belief that the higher being will be the one to make the choice of when."

"So what can I do?" Stan asks. "Can people really change? Can I?"

The truth is that our finest moments are most likely to occur when we are feeling deeply uncomfortable, unhappy, or unfulfilled. For it is only in such moments, propelled by our discomfort, that we are likely to step out of our ruts and start searching for different ways or truer answers.

—M. Scott Peck

Suggestions for Achieving Acceptance and Peace

Questions to Consider

- Why do you want to "let go"?
- Are you avoiding a review of your past? If so, why?
- Can you bring closure to unresolved issues? See "Is It Too Late to Make Amends?" (page 137).
- Can you accept that you cannot change the past—only the present?
- Are you tired of your life as it is now? If so, why?
- What actions can you take to address these reasons for unhappiness? Some reasons for unhappiness may include:

  Lack of close relationships with others—if so, explore ways to deepen relationships; perhaps call or write loved ones or old friends and share how much you care for and value them. Take the first step and feel a sense of happiness at reaching out, regardless of how the person responds.

  Physical discomfort—if so, talk with your health care team about ways to improve your comfort.

  Unhappiness with your living arrangements—if so, what can you do to make your surroundings more to your liking?

- Are you hoping to avoid becoming dependent on others? If so, see "I Don't Want to Be a Burden . . ." (page 33).
- Are you afraid of the unknown?

  Do you fear something specific, or do you fear simply not knowing what will happen?

  If you fear something specific, is there someone you can talk with about your concerns, like a chaplain, a social worker, a nurse, a spiritual leader, or another counselor?

  If you fear the uncertainty of not knowing what the future holds, look back on your life, on other periods of uncertainty, and recall what you did to cope during those times. What gives you your strength? Can you draw on that now?

- Are you impatient to reach an afterlife? If so, review your spiritual teachings and practices. Are you supposed to receive something simply because you ask or pray for it? Or does your faith reflect an acceptance that a higher being ultimately decides the timing of such things?

- What does *letting go* mean to you?

  Does *letting go* mean passing within a specific length of time? If so, why have you specified a time frame?

  Does *letting go* mean accepting the time and situation as it is, without expectation?

- What does the word *peace* mean to you?

  What can you do to achieve this?

  Are the people around you—your loved ones and others—accepting of your situation and supportive of your desire to achieve peace? If not, what can be done to help them achieve acceptance and peace?

  Can you ask a spiritual leader, a social worker, or a hospice nurse to help them address their issues?

- Is this a good moment?

  If not, what needs to change to make it a good moment?

  If it is, breathe in, savor it, and exhale. Enjoy this moment, and what other moments may follow.

  Live a good life now. Live a good moment now.

Why Me?
❃ Why Am I Being Punished? ❃
Reconciling Mortality with Your Religious Beliefs

Irma and Harry

"GOD IS GOING TO GRANT ME A MIRACLE," Irma declares, propped amidst a pile of pillows on her king-size bed. The seven ladies gathered around the bed all nod in agreement. One of the ladies lays a hand on Irma's arm. "Amen . . . Amen. And we're going to pray with you, Sister Irma. God will decide you are worthy of His grace. He will not take you." As the fervent prayer commences, I slip out of the room and join Irma's husband, Harry, in the kitchen.

"What do you think?" Harry asks, pulling out a chair, inviting me to sit. "Is she going to get better?"

Irma's body is riddled with cancer, but her mind remains clear, even with the high doses of pain medication required to keep her comfortable. "I don't know," I say as I settle into the chair. "I can tell you how she's doing now."

Most of my visits proceed like this one. I ask Irma how she's feeling, if anything concerns her. I ask about her symptoms, if she's comfortable, adjusting her dose of pain medication, if needed. At the end of each visit, she tells me, "God is going to grant me a miracle." Then the ladies from the church arrive for a few hours of prayer, as if to chase away any thoughts that end-of-life care is needed. "God is testing you, Sister Irma. But He will grant you a miracle. You will be saved. You will be cured."

The weeks pass and Irma, now gaunt, continues to prop herself up in bed and pray fervently with the ladies of the church, her bony hands in theirs, her head bowed. I notice that one lady sits away from the bed. When hands are joined, she hesitates. Then one day she doesn't come. "Child care problems," explains one of the ladies. A week later another stops coming. The following week, two more. As Irma grows thinner, the prayer circle grows smaller. Finally, only Harry remains to sit at her bedside and pray.

I ask Irma if having congregation members pray with her is important to her. "Oh, yes," she replies, "but they're all busy."

"Would you like me to call the pastor to ask if he can put the word out that you'd like people to pray with you?"

She shakes her head. "Pastor calls once a week. He tells me they're praying for me, for a miracle, at church."

When she continues to decline, Harry becomes unable to manage her care at home. They choose a nice care facility near their home and church. Again, I ask if they'd like me to call the pastor, to let him know of the change, that Irma could use some extra support.

"We told him," Harry says. "He said he'd ask the congregation to visit. Said he'd stop by, too."

When I check in with the staff at the care facility, I learn that the pastor has come to visit. "He didn't stay too long," the nurse's aide shares. "He prayed with her, asking God for a miracle. Then he hurried out. He looked pretty uncomfortable, too."

I step into Irma's room. By now, she is emaciated. Skin stretches over bone. "How are you?" I ask as I pull a chair close to her bed.

She blinks, but makes no other response. I lower the bed rail and take hold of her bony hand. Her fingers curl around mine. "Will you pray with me?" she asks in a hoarse whisper.

I lower my head. At the end of her prayers, I gaze at her skeleton-like body, which has defied all her doctors' predictions.

"I'm still alive," she says weakly. "Maybe I'm going to get my miracle after all."

I offer a gentle smile.

"Will you help me roll to my side? I'm too weak even to do that for myself, and I'm so thin it hurts to lie in one position for more than a little while."

I ease her to her side, propping soft pillows where bone meets bone: at her knees, her ankles, beneath her arm as it rests across her ribs. "I heard that the pastor came to see you," I say, settling once more in the chair, my eyes again level with her. "Has anyone else from your church been by?"

She blinks and turns away. "They're all busy. Young children. Church activities. Who has extra time these days?"

Once, before Irma had progressed to this state, congregation members found hours several times each week to sit with her to pray for a miracle. And now, as Irma hovers near death, they do not come.

"How do you feel about them not being here?"

She blinks several times, but does not answer.

"I'm very worried about you," I confess.

Irma looks at me, startled.

"I can't help but wonder: How will you feel about your God if you're not granted the miracle you pray for? How will you feel about yourself?"

Irma draws a deep breath. She stares at me. Finally, she whispers, "Am I going to die?"

"I think it's very likely that you will die very soon."

She swallows. Her gaze flits away from mine. "Then God is punishing me. I haven't been a good enough follower. That's why the people of the church have stopped coming. God isn't going to grant me a miracle." A tear slides down her cheek.

"What do your scriptures teach about death, about an afterlife?" I ask.

"We join God and Jesus in heaven."

"Do you think that's a reward or a punishment from God?"

"It's a reward!" she declares, frowning that such a question would need to be asked.

"What do your scriptures teach about miracles?"

For a long time she stares at me. Finally, she answers. "That God has the power to grant them. That these acts can defy all laws of nature. God has that power."

"I look at you, Irma, and I see a miracle. I see someone who has defied what every doctor predicted. You have lived longer than anyone would have ever thought possible. And I have to wonder: Is that a miracle? Is your being alive something for us all to learn from? The congregation at your church, people like me, the doctors, and, most of all, you. Has God given all of us, through you—by granting you the strength to continue as long as you have—a chance to learn something deeply important?"

"But if I still die, how is that a miracle?"

"We all die, Irma. Saints and sinners alike. None of us are granted immortality. Death is not a punishment."

"Then what's the miracle?"

"I wouldn't presume to know the answer to that. What I *can* tell you is what I think I, and others perhaps, have had the chance to learn."

"What is that?"

"The congregation at your church—maybe they've been given a chance to explore what faith really means to them. Is faith a belief that God will give us what we ask for, or is it accepting that God knows things we cannot? To put it another way, that God might have other plans for us.

"As you became weaker, the people at your church had a difficult time being around you. I think they were afraid. I think we all, to some extent, feel that illness and death happen only to other people. Seeing that even you, a member of their congregation, a deeply religious woman, could succumb, rocked their belief that somehow they were exempt. If God could allow someone like you to be stricken with cancer, then it could strike them, too. Perhaps that realization was just too much for many of them to cope with, so they just stopped coming. In doing so, they were able to cling to some degree of denial about their own mortality."

"I'd wondered that myself," she confesses. "My sister said the same thing you did. She doesn't think much of the people in my church."

"So maybe you've given them a chance to learn. The longer you live, the more times they hear your name from the pulpit. 'Sister Irma needs our prayers.' Maybe they're asking themselves: 'Why aren't we praying with Sister Irma? And what is it, truly, to be saved?'"

"Maybe . . . And what about you? You said maybe I'd offered some kind of miracle, some kind of lesson to you, too."

I smile. "At least once a day a family member takes me aside and asks, 'How long?' How much longer will their loved one live? This is what I tell them: I've been doing this long enough to know that I don't know, that the body tells us one thing, but the spirit, perhaps even more than the body, determines when we pass.

"Spending these last months with you, I'm reminded of just how true that is." I cup her hand in my palms. "I will meet other people like you, Irma, people who wonder, 'Is death a punishment from God? Have I failed Him in some way?' I will remember you, and what you taught me. And these lessons, I hope, will help them. *You* will help them.

"Maybe God isn't punishing you, Irma. Maybe you're living this long, even though your body should have given out long ago, because you have the inner strength to teach others."

Tears flow down her cheeks. "And what lesson does He offer me? For all this, what's my lesson? What is my miracle?"

I hold her hand, but say nothing. She waits, then smiles and says, "I'm going to close my eyes now. I'm going to think about what that answer might be."

The life I touch for good or ill will touch another life, and that in turn another, until who knows where the trembling stops or in what far place my touch will be felt.

—Frederick Buechner

To fly, we have to have resistance.

—Maya Lin

Questions for Exploring Your View of the Spiritual Meaning of Death

- What are your beliefs about illness and death as a part of life and the cycle of nature?
- What are your beliefs about the purpose of life?
- How do you see your life and death within the context of your beliefs about the purpose of life?
- What are your beliefs about the journey of the soul or spirit?
- Do you believe in an afterlife? If so, what form does that afterlife take? What entitles a soul to attain this afterlife? How do your thoughts and actions affect this passage?
- Do you feel, even within the limitations and challenges of your illness, that you are living your beliefs?
- If not, what actions do you need to take to achieve spiritual peace?
- Within the teachings of your faith, is it possible that death might be the ultimate form of healing?

We Always Thought We'd Have More Time . . .

*Realizing Dreams and Appreciating the Choices
You Have Made*

Galen and His Family

"WE ALWAYS THOUGHT WE'D HAVE MORE TIME," Galen says, his voice trailing off. Mary, his wife, reaches for his hand as they sit together on their sofa.

"We always planned to travel," she adds, "after the kids were grown. But for some reason, we always put it off . . ."

Galen stares, unseeing, at the carpet, and I wonder what other dreams remain unrealized for him, for both of them.

For this I have no easy answers, no soothing words, no medicines. I cannot turn the clock back to the last time—months ago, perhaps years ago—when they said, "We'll do it later . . . We have time." What they have is this moment: four months, maybe five. I make a note: *Wanted to travel.*

Later I call their son, Colin, who lives about an hour's drive away. Galen has granted permission for me to talk with his family, and placed no restrictions on what is shared. I update Colin on his dad's health, and ask about his parents' travel dreams.

"They always meant to. Something always came up. They'd add something to the house—the deck, a hot tub, things like that. And they enjoyed all those things. A few years ago, my sister, brother, and I decided to pool our money and surprise them with the airfare. But with kids of our own, we couldn't afford to pay for the whole thing. Money's tight for all of us. Now I wish we had, somehow.

"Anyway, they were really touched when we offered, but said they couldn't accept it. By then, I think travel had become something they just talked about. They'd watch the travel channel and get a real kick out of it. They could sit in their own home and not have to go to all the trouble of dragging suitcases around to see these things."

As I listen, an idea takes shape. Three weeks later, at the end of their usual morning call, Colin asks his dad if he's up for a visit later that day. When Galen responds with an enthusiastic, "You bet," Colin urges his father to take a nap. "So I don't wear you out. And tell Mom I'll bring something for dinner, so she doesn't need to cook."

That evening Colin, and Colin's sister and brother, along with their spouses and children, stand together and ring the bell. Mary opens the door. Her eyes widen. Her hands fly to her open mouth. "Galen . . . Galen . . . They're all here!" Tears flow and hugs abound. The family has not all gathered together for a few years, as all but Colin have moved to other states.

From Colin's minivan they bring in dish after dish of foods from Paris, Mexico, Hawaii, and all the other places Galen and Mary had hoped to visit. Squeezed together in Galen and Mary's living room, they play travel videos and, as a family, journey together around the world.

"I always wanted to see these places," Galen says, wiping a stray tear, his other arm wrapped around a grandson. "But this is better. Much better. I get to enjoy it with all of you."

Harriet and Gene

"Can you come later?" Harriet asks. "After one? Our favorite soap opera is on from noon to one. We hate to miss it."

For the next month I plan visits around the angst of *Days of Our Lives*. When I ask Harriet and Gene how they're faring, more often than not I hear about the woes of the soap opera heroine and her latest challenge with love and life.

In their eighties, Harriet and Gene manage on a very small income, with every penny stretched to the limit. Their one luxury is to watch their old console television from morning until night, completely enthralled by the lives of others. Years ago, even before Harriet became ill, they stopped venturing out, and when the senior service began delivering groceries, they no longer needed to go out at all. Soon, they stopped opening the curtains. "Casts a glare on the TV," Gene explained.

One day, when Gene is looking particularly tired, having taken on all the household chores, I ask if they have any friends living nearby who might be willing to help.

"Everybody's old, like us," Gene says. "There's this couple we used to play cards with. Live two houses down, across the street. They come by with a casserole now and then. Real nice people."

"Anybody else?" I ask. Gene and Harriet name a few friends, all living within a few blocks. "But we haven't seen them for a while."

"Would you like to?"

"That might be nice, but I'm not up to entertaining," Harriet says, taking a sip of tea. "And besides, I'd miss my shows."

One afternoon Harriet shares that her favorite soap opera heroine is celebrating her wedding anniversary. I suppress a smile of amazement that any soap opera heroine remains married for more than a year, and instead ask Harriet and Gene how long they've been married.

They look at each other, brows furrowed, trying to remember. Finally, Gene says, "It's coming up on sixty years. I just came out of the navy, and we got married pretty soon after that."

"You sure?" Harriet asks.

Gene nods. "Yep. Came out in '35. Met you that same month. Your brother introduced us."

"You remember all that?"

"You bet I do. You were wearing this light blue dress, and I remember thinking I'd better be quick or somebody else was going to snatch you up."

"I think I remember you being pretty handsome, too."

From the television, some drama plays out, but neither Harriet nor Gene notice. "When were you married?" I ask. "Do you remember the date?"

"It was August," Gene says. "Hot as hell. I remember that now. I got a little stuck there for a minute, but it was August. August of '35."

"My goodness," Harriet says. "You do remember." Then she turns to me. "We have our own anniversary coming up."

Silently, I count off the months until August. It's not likely that Harriet will be alive. If she is, she will not be feeling well. She will not be able to sit in her living room and enjoy a moment like this. But I say nothing. Instead, after my visit I call my next appointment and arrange a later time. Then I dash to a grocery store to buy a simple bouquet of flowers, sparkling cider, and a small cake. I hurry back and knock on the door. "Happy anniversary!" I cheer as Gene, opening the door, squints at the bright light. "Why not celebrate today?" I ask.

Gene and Harriet stare at me. Then both their faces break into wide grins. On my later visits, I arrive to find the television off. And as I sit beside Harriet, she leans close and shares, not the latest television tragedy, but the stories that she and Gene are rediscovering of the life they shared, the little things that, now, they laugh about . . . Life. Their life, together.

Yesterday is but a dream, and tomorrow is but a vision. But today well lived makes every yesterday a dream of happiness and every tomorrow a vision of hope. Look well, therefore, to this day.

—Kálidása

The best time to plant a tree is twenty years ago. The next-best time is now.

—Chinese Proverb

Suggestions for Realizing Dreams

- Consider unrealized dreams. Is there a way to realize the spirit of these dreams, given the situation? Can your loved ones help?
- Celebrate now.
- Don't wait to have meaningful conversations.
- Ask loved ones to visit now, while you can enjoy their company.
- Reflect on the choices you made, all that you enjoyed in lieu of realizing the dream. Recognize the value of what you chose.

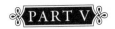

PART V

For Loved Ones and Caregivers: Sharing the Final Days

This section offers information that may be especially helpful for loved ones and caregivers. To better understand and prepare for the issues presented in this section, consider reading these chapters before the final days.

In this section you'll learn how to care for someone in the final days. You'll find information about physical changes that may occur, and what these changes mean. You'll learn how to keep your loved one comfortable, and how to recognize if she's comfortable, even if she can't tell you how she feels. You'll also discover what you can do at the time of passing to honor your loved one and create a special memory, if you choose.

How Do We Keep Her Comfortable?
Giving Medication When Your Loved One Can No Longer Swallow
Recognizing If Your Loved One Is in Pain
Preventing Discomfort

How Do I Let Go?
Saying Good-bye: Helping Your Loved One Achieve Peace

How Will We Know When the End Is Near?
Changes You May See
Understanding What These Changes Mean

I Want to Be with Her When She Passes . . .
Meeting Your Loved One's Needs—and Yours—in the Final Days
Ideas to Create a Peaceful Environment

I Want My Last Memory to Be a Good Memory . . .
What to Do at the Time of Death
Ideas for Honoring and Caring for Your Loved One at the Time of Death

How Do We Keep Her Comfortable?

Giving Medication When Your Loved One Can No Longer Swallow
Recognizing If Your Loved One Is in Pain
Preventing Discomfort

Miriam and Her Family

"IT'S GETTING TO BE REALLY DIFFICULT TO wake Mom for her medication. She's really slow to swallow. And when we ask if she's comfortable, she's not really able to answer," says Warren, the eldest of Miriam's three grown children who have gathered to care for her in her final days. "What do we do?" he asks. "How do we keep her comfortable?"

I gaze at each of the siblings. On their faces I see anxiety, but also earnestness, a desire to do the best they can for their mom. "As we get closer to dying, in general, we become less responsive," I point out. "We sleep most of the time, and we're very difficult to arouse. Later, we may not be able to be awakened, or, if we are, we may not be able to swallow. It sounds like your mom is at or near this point."

The family nods and I continue. "One of the challenges is how to give your mom the medications she needs to stay comfortable. Another challenge is how to recognize if she's comfortable when she's not able to communicate her needs."

"That's what we need to know," says Miriam's daughter, Tammy.

"First, let's look at the list of your mom's medications. At this point we have to decide which of these are needed to keep her comfortable. The rest we eliminate. Next we figure out how to get these medications into her system in the least invasive way. Finally, I'll share with you how to determine if your mom is comfortable when she's not able to communicate. I'll also give you some information about what you can do to prevent discomfort."

"That sounds helpful," Warren says.

I call the physician and update him on the situation. He decides which medications to discontinue, which to continue to maintain comfort, and how best to administer each medication, given that Miriam can no longer safely swallow.

HOW TO GIVE MEDICINE SAFELY: TIMED-RELEASE MEDICINE

Let's start with the timed-release, long-acting pain medication. We run some serious risks if we continue to attempt to give this pill by mouth. Because she can't consistently swallow, she could choke on a pill. Or she could bite down on it or it could simply lie in her mouth and dissolve. If that happened, the medicine would be released into her system in one large dose, rather than over time. So to get this timed-release medication safely into her system, we need to choose another route.

One option would be to start an IV and infuse the medication directly. But this would require you to learn how to manage an IV line here in the home. It's fairly technical. Everything must be kept sterile. The line has to be managed to ensure that it remains patent and doesn't clot. On top of everything else you have to learn and do in these last days, managing an IV in the home is a lot to take on.

Another option would be to switch to a patch that delivers pain medication through the skin. It works quite well for certain doses of medication. Unfortunately, the lowest available dose of the patch would be too much for your mom right now. If her dosage increases, we'll definitely want to consider the patch.

If her dose were really low, we'd simply use the short-acting medicine that can be placed under her tongue, and give it every four hours. Unfortunately, if we converted all her pain medicine to the short-acting liquid, she'd need more than could be safely placed under her tongue. We'd run the risk of her choking. A little is okay, but too much is risky.

So the best choice, at this point, will be to give the timed-release pain medicine rectally. I know this isn't something anyone really wants to do. But it's the best available option to keep her free of pain. Some families are really uncomfortable with this. It's not easy to think about doing this for someone else. It's an invasion of privacy—but it's also a way to give her comfort at a time when she depends on others to care for her.

She takes the long-acting medicine every twelve hours. So you'd need to do this only twice a day for these last days. You simply put some lubricant on the capsule and, wearing a glove, insert it in the rectum.

If two of you can work together, it may be easier for your mom. Together you can gently roll her to her side. One of you can then help steady her in that position while the other inserts the medicine.

How to Give the Medicine Safely: Short-Acting, Immediate-Release Medicine

It's a little easier to give medicine that's not timed-release. In many cases, this medicine comes in a very concentrated, liquid form, so she doesn't have to swallow it. It's simply absorbed from under her tongue or in the pocket of her cheek.

I'll give you a special, extra-small syringe that has an open end. There's no needle. It's calibrated so that you can draw up the right amount of medication. And because it's small, it's fairly easy to slip gently into her mouth, along her cheek or under her tongue.

You want to be careful, though, that the medicine doesn't just trickle down the back of her throat. Maybe raise her head a little, or turn her head to the side while you're giving it. Afterward, just wash the syringe in a little dish soap. Treat it as you would a spoon.

You can give certain short-acting pills this way, too. You'll just crush or dissolve them first. One technique that works well is to use that small syringe without the needle. Take the plunger out and place the pill inside. Then, put the plunger back in. Pour some hot water into a small bowl. Draw up a little water into the syringe, no more than about a half a milliliter. Gently shake the syringe. This helps dissolve the pill. Let it sit for a few minutes before you give it. Then gently ease the syringe under her tongue or into the pocket of her cheek and administer the medicine.

This technique works well for the medicine your mom is on now. Unfortunately, it doesn't work for all short-acting pills. Some are too big for this technique. Some can't be crushed or dissolved. So if we do add any new medication, we'll need to talk about each pill on a case-by-case basis.

How Will We Know if She's in Pain?

Given that your mom can't tell you how she feels, either with words or gestures, you'll want to be able to recognize when she's having pain or is uncomfortable.

Whether we are conscious or not, our facial expressions reveal how we feel. Look at your mom's face. Is her brow furrowed? Does her expression appear tense, maybe even frowning? If you see these signs, give some of that concentrated liquid immediate-release pain medicine. Wait about an hour. Then take another good look at her face. Does she appear relaxed? Is the frown gone? Is her forehead relaxed? Those signs tell us that a person is comfortable.

Also, listen. Is she making sounds? Sometimes people vocalize. It might be a steady tone or a murmur. This may not mean she's in pain. When someone *is* in pain, that sound is usually a fairly clear moan. If she's making sounds, look at her face as well to help guide you.

Sometimes people will be very comfortable at rest, but may experience pain when they're turned, so you'll want to pay close attention when you reposition her. If she consistently shows signs of discomfort when she's turned, it's a good idea to start giving the immediate-release pain medicine *before* you turn her to prevent discomfort. Just slip a little under her tongue, wait about thirty minutes, and then turn her.

Preventing Discomfort: Positioning

There are many other things you can do for your mom besides medication to help keep her comfortable. Earlier, I mentioned repositioning her. When we lie in one place for a long time, we get stiff. What you'll want to do is gently reposition her every couple of hours. Tip her onto her side, then her back, and then to her other side. Tuck extra pillows along her back and thigh to support her when she's on her side. Basically, you want to place her in what looks like a comfortable position. Make sure her knees and ankles aren't bone-on-bone and that her arms are supported. Use extra pillows if you need to. Make sure her back and hips are aligned, and that her head looks comfortably propped up. When you finish, stand back and ask yourself: Would I be comfortable resting like this?

Since you'll need to turn her around the clock, you might want to take shifts so that you're each able to rest.

PREVENTING DISCOMFORT: DRY MOUTH AND DRY EYES

Another possible source of discomfort is a dry mouth, especially if she's breathing through her mouth. Because she's not alert, you don't want to put any food or beverage in her mouth that she would need to swallow.

You can keep her comfortable by periodically moistening her mouth with a swab. I'll give you some. The swab looks a bit like a lollipop, except there's a small sponge at the end. Just dampen it lightly in water, tap off any excess, and gently swab the inside of her mouth. You don't want so much water on the sponge that it drips down the back of her throat and causes her to choke. Also, be sure to use water—not mouthwash or anything with lemon or glycerin. These will cause the mouth to dry out more. The goal is to moisten the mouth a little, so she stays comfortable. You can also apply a little balm or ointment to her lips to keep them moist, too.

Also, she might rest with her eyes open. If so, her eyes might become a little dry. You can place a few drops of over-the-counter artificial tears in her eyes every few hours. That will help.

PREVENTING DISCOMFORT: FEVER

She might begin to run a fever, which could be caused by a variety of reasons. Regardless of the cause, in general, we're not uncomfortable until our temperature goes above 100 degrees Fahrenheit (38°C). Since

I try to be as noninvasive as possible, rather than use a thermometer, I touch the forehead or the chest to give me the best sense of the person's core temperature. Check your Mom like this periodically. If she feels warm, draw back all but the sheet and apply a cool cloth to her forehead, refreshing it frequently. If she continues to feel warm, or begins to feel hot, add cool cloths to the armpits, abdomen, and groin and change them frequently, or gently wipe her arms, abdomen, and legs with a cool cloth. You could also draw back the sheet and direct a fan, set at low speed, to blow gently across the skin.

If she still feels hot, the next question would be: Does she look uncomfortable? If not, then continue with the cool cloths and fan. If she *does* look uncomfortable, then it's time to consider acetaminophen suppositories. But recall that fever in the final days has a variety of causes. Acetaminophen works for only some of those causes, and if it does work, she is likely to sweat—a lot. That might require a change of sheets and a sponge bath, which might be even more uncomfortable than the fever. Also, if the acetaminophen does work, you'll need to continue to insert it rectally every four hours to keep the fever down. So it's a good idea to try cool cloths and fans first, and consider acetaminophen suppositories only if she looks uncomfortable.

Should We Give IV Fluids?

If your mom was alert and active, and her inability to swallow resulted from a tumor, or a muscle or nerve disorder, providing fluids or artificial nutrition could add weeks or months to her life. But your mom is within days of passing, not because she isn't getting nutrition or fluids, but because of her disease process.

We can give IV fluids; in some cases, such as delirium occurring in the final days, a small volume of IV fluid, infused very slowly, might be helpful to keep her comfortable. But, in general, giving IV fluids in the final days or hours isn't a good idea. As the body is beginning to shut down, it has a remarkable way of protecting itself. Remember when your mom's appetite began to decline and she wasn't able to eat certain foods, like meats or large meals? That was her body saying it couldn't process those foods anymore.

As we get closer to dying, our kidneys begin to shut down. We aren't able to eliminate normal volumes of fluid from our system anymore. As part of this process, we lose our ability to swallow, to take in liquids or other nutrition that we would be unable to process. So if we were to override this natural protection by inserting an IV line and forcing fluids into her that she wouldn't otherwise take in, her body won't be able to process and eliminate all that extra fluid.

At this time, the heart is also beginning its decline. It's no longer able to function as well as it once did. Extra fluid would place an additional burden on her declining heart. As the heart becomes unable to keep up, that extra fluid will begin to seep into places it's not supposed to go. It might cause her legs to swell. Most likely, though, it will fill her lungs and her death would result from something much like drowning. But I'm glad you asked. Caring for someone in her final days isn't something many people have experience with. It's important to ask questions, and to understand, rather than wonder later if there was something more you could have done.

You love her and you want to do the right thing. By understanding this process and knowing what you can do to support her, you'll ensure that she's comfortable and at peace, and you'll be more at peace, too.

We don't receive wisdom; we must discover it for ourselves after a journey no one can take for us or spare us.

—Marcel Proust

KEEPING YOUR LOVED ONE COMFORTABLE IN THE FINAL DAYS
Nonverbal Signs of Pain
- Furrowed brow
- Grimace
- Moaning at rest or with turns or care

- Restlessness (may also be a sign of anxiety or emotional distress)

Preventing Discomfort

- Review the medication list with your hospice nurse or health care provider. Discuss possible changes and how best to give each medication. Write down the new instructions.
- Gently reposition her every two hours, using pillows for support.
- If her mouth is dry, dampen a swab and gently wipe the inside of her mouth every two to four hours. Discontinue this if secretions build up in the mouth and congestion occurs. See "How Will We Know When the End Is Near?" (page 170).
- Apply lip balm or ointment to her lips every two to four hours.
- If her eyes remain open, apply artificial tears every two to four hours.
- Maintain a quiet, peaceful environment.
- Avoid shining bright light in her eyes. If you bring her outside, place sunglasses on her, or position her with her face in the shade.
- If signs of pain occur during turns or when changing disposable underwear, medicate with immediate-release pain medication thirty minutes to one hour before turns and incontinence care.
- Minimize personal hygiene care during the final days.
  Perform minimal bathing only.
  Discontinue tooth brushing.
  Discontinue or decrease frequency of facial shaving.
- For more information about pain medication, see "Appendix C: Common Pain Medications" (page 216).

❊ How Do I Let Go? ❊
Saying Good-bye: Helping Your Loved One Achieve Peace

Wendell and Jill

"Daddy?" Jill says quietly as she leans close to the bed, holding her father's hand.

Wendell opens one eye briefly and attempts to smile.

Jill settles on the edge of the bed. "How are you feeling today?"

Wendell doesn't answer.

Jill turns to me. "How's he doing? He seems pretty sleepy today. Did you just give him extra medicine? Is that why he's so sleepy?"

I shake my head. "We haven't given him any additional medication that would cause sedation. He's getting the same doses he's been getting for the past five days."

"He was more awake yesterday . . . Daddy? Do you want to say hello to Bret? He's here . . ."

She waits. Wendell doesn't open his eyes.

After Wendell's diagnosis with incurable cancer, his daughter Jill took a leave of absence from her job, postponed her wedding to Bret, and moved back into her old room at her parents' house. Her arrival brought a surge of energy and joy to Wendell's life.

Ten days ago, as the cancer advanced and he developed new pain, he came to the hospice house for adjustment of his medications. Within two days, he was his old self again—comfortable, joking with the staff, beaming as his daughter stepped into the room, drawing her in with a big bear hug and an eager smile. Plans were made for him to return home again. Then he began to decline. It was as if the energy he felt during his daughter's visits vanished the moment she left the room. Weariness settled over his face. He slept more. His skin paled. He stopped eating and drinking.

Over the next three days, we saw even more decline. His time with his daughter no longer gave him a burst of energy; rather, it became a difficult struggle as he attempted to remain awake, alert, smiling, sitting up, pretending that nothing had changed.

Today when she stepped into the room, Wendell did not sit up. He did not reach for her. He couldn't.

"Daddy?" Jill waits. Then she turns to me. "What's happening? Why isn't he getting up? Why isn't he like he was?"

I kneel beside her. "He can hear you, but his energy level is declining. He's getting weaker."

Jill turns to her father. She shakes her head and clutches his hand. "You can't get worse, Daddy. You just can't." Her voice breaks. "I need you. I need you," she sobs.

Wendell attempts to open his eyes. He lifts his hand a few inches off the bed, toward Jill, but his strength fails and his hand falls back onto the blanket. He closes his eyes. A tear falls across his cheek.

I lay my arm around Jill's shoulders. I glance at Bret, who stands on the other side of the bed, hands hanging awkwardly at his sides, his expression haunted as he watches the woman he loves feel such pain.

"There has to be something we can do," Jill pleads. "You can't leave me, Daddy. I need you. Don't let go!"

Again Wendell struggles to open his eyes, to speak, to reach for her. But he cannot.

"Jill, there is something you can do for your dad . . . Every day we've watched how his face lights up when you arrive, how happy he is when you're here. If he could, if he had a choice, I believe he would never leave you.

"Even now, when he can't speak, I see the anguish in his face because he can't comfort you. He can't promise you that things will be all right. No matter how much he wants things to be different, he can't change this."

She gazes at her father, her chest rising and falling with deep, shaking breaths.

My arm tightens around her shoulders. "I believe that you, more than anyone else, can give him peace."

She turns to me. Then she looks again at her dad as he lies in the bed. Tears stream down her face. For a long while, we sit together beside Wendell's bed.

Then Jill leans toward the bed. Her lips brush Wendell's forehead and her hands cradle his. "I love you, Daddy. I love you, and I will miss you . . . I'll miss you so much—but I'll be all right. I'll hold you here in my heart. You will always be with me . . ."

I love you.
I forgive you.
Please forgive me.
Thank you.

—*Adapted from the traditional Hawaiian teachings of* Ho'oponopono, *meaning*
"To Make Right"

SUGGESTIONS FOR SAYING GOOD-BYE

In preparing to say good-bye, consider:

- What are some of the most important things you have learned from your loved one?
- What have you learned about courage and strength from your loved one?
- How will these lessons help you as you grieve?
- In what other positive ways will these lessons influence how you live after your loved one has passed?
- What do you want to thank him for?
- Are there unresolved issues for which you want to ask forgiveness? If so, can you ask for forgiveness? Can you accept that your loved one would grant that forgiveness, even if he isn't able to communicate?
- Do you believe that your loved one would ask forgiveness for his actions, if he were able to? If so, can you offer your forgiveness, even though your loved one has not asked for it?
- Even though you will likely feel great sadness and loss, do you feel that, somehow, you'll be okay? (If you don't feel you'll be able to

cope, seek additional support from your community, such as your spiritual community, your other loved ones, the hospice team, or others.)

+ Even if your loved one may no longer be able to respond, it's very likely he can still hear you. Can you offer your loved one peace and comfort by saying thank you, by asking for and accepting forgiveness? Can you find and share a sense of inner peace? Can you say good-bye?

How Will We Know When the End Is Near?

Changes You May See
Understanding What These Changes Mean

Bob and Beverly

"**Should we talk in the other room?**" Beverly asks as I arrive at her home.

I turn to Bob, her husband, who lies in a hospital bed nearby, in the center of the family's living room. He is completely unresponsive. Earlier, on the phone, Beverly had shared that Bob's only reaction in the last twenty-four hours has been to bite down on the swab as she gently moistened his mouth.

"It's up to you," I say. "I believe he can hear us."

"Really?"

I nod. "There have been studies done on survivors of near-death experiences. Often they can repeat what was said by paramedics and emergency medical staff. My coworkers and I could all share hundreds of stories about how people who are as nonresponsive as Bob appear to hear and understand."

"How can you tell?"

"Sometimes it's subtle, like a small facial change. Sometimes we'll have a family member who can't be with a loved one in the final days. We'll hold the phone close so that the faraway family member can say good-bye. Even in people who are nonresponsive, we'll see tiny changes— eyelids fluttering, tiny movements of their lips, little things—enough to tell us that they, in some way, are aware of their loved one's voice."

"So Bob can hear us?"

"I believe he can."

She turns to Bob. "That would be nice . . . to be able to talk to him, to know that he can hear me, even if he can't respond." She moves to stand beside the bed.

"How long have you been married?" I ask.

She smiles. "Fifteen years. We were both divorced. Our kids introduced us. Neither of us ever thought we'd get married again." She smoothes a thick lock of graying hair from Bob's forehead. "He's the best thing that ever happened to me."

"I suspect he feels the same way about you."

Her gaze lingers on Bob. "Let's talk here," she says, reaching for a tissue. "I want to be with him. I want him to know what's going on." She settles in the chair beside the bed and I sit nearby, on the couch.

"How long," she asks, reaching for Bob's hand. "How long do you think he has? His kids want to be here. Mine do, too." Her voice breaks. "I want to be beside him."

I look at Bob, at the color of his face. Then I stand and approach the bed. I watch him breathe, listening to the rhythm, the slow in and out. My gaze wanders around the room, lingering on the photos of their blended family, of their wedding, of their life together. In one photo Bob stands on a riverbank holding his catch. He is smiling, not at the camera, or at the gleaming, silver fish he holds, but at the grinning boy who stands beside him, struggling to hold aloft his own catch—easily twice the size of Bob's.

Bob's breathing pauses. I count the seconds. He appears peaceful, comfortable. I wait. The breathing resumes. "Bob," I say in a very soft voice, "you're going to feel my hands, very gently, at your wrists." I feel for the pulses at his wrists. Both are fairly strong. His hands are warm.

"You're going to feel me gently place a stethoscope against your chest." I warm the stethoscope on my palm, then slip it inside his pajama top. His lungs sound clear, without congestion.

"Next you're going to feel me gently drawing aside the covers around your knees. Then you'll feel my hands on your knees." I place my palms on his knees; both are cool. I bend and look closely at their coloring. They're pale, but I see no other discoloration. I replace the quilt. I glance at Bob's face. He shows no reaction to my touch. I proceed.

"Next you'll feel me draw back the covers around your feet. Then you'll feel me gently touch your feet." Like his knees, his feet are both cool. I feel only a faint pulse on each foot. I bend to look at the soles. On the pad of his right sole I see a purplish, blotchy discoloration. I motion Beverly to come close. "Do you see that purplish discoloration?" I ask.

She nods.

"That's mottling," I say, drawing the covers back over Bob's feet. "In a moment I'll tell you what that means."

Beverly resumes her place beside Bob and I settle again on the couch. "I'll write down what I'm about to share with you, about what signs you might see as Bob is getting closer."

"Thank you," Beverly says. "There's been so much to learn and do."

"It's a difficult job, caring for a loved one. You're doing a great job."

She smiles and squeezes Bob's hand. "The kids help. And Bob helps, in his own way."

She continues to gaze at Bob, and I sit quietly, not intruding on her moment. What comes next—the signs she might see when Bob is close to passing—represents another step for her and her family, another passage, the last passage.

With her hand holding Bob's, she turns to me.

"I've been doing this long enough to know that I don't know exactly how, exactly when," I say gently. "Each of us does this in our own way, in our own time. Sometimes we see many physical signs, and sometimes only a few. I've learned, however, that people seem to choose their time. Some choose to be alone. Some choose to wait for loved ones to arrive. Through it all, I communicate with the person making the journey. I'll tell him if I've called his loved ones, who I've talked to, if that person is coming in, and, if so, when she'll arrive. Ultimately, the person will make his own choice of when to let go and leave us.

"You saw me watch him. I was also listening to the way he's breathing. You may have noticed the pauses in his breathing. Right now the pauses are lasting about twenty seconds and occur every few minutes. As time goes by, you may notice the pauses becoming longer and more frequent.

"Right now he's breathing easily, without effort. Later you might notice some congestion, a slight gurgling coming from the back of his throat. As we get closer to dying we lose the ability to cough and swallow. When that happens, secretions sometimes build up in the back of the throat. Generally, if it's mild, these secretions, this gurgling, doesn't cause any discomfort for the person. It's usually more troubling for other people to listen to these sounds.

"If he does begin to sound congested, you'll want to turn him onto his side and raise the head of the bed a little. That will keep the secretions from pooling in his throat. You'll also want to stop moistening his mouth with the damp swabs. If the congestion worsens, call us. We'll call the doctor for a medication that might help relieve that."

"What about suctioning?" she asks. "Would that help?"

"Generally, suctioning only makes it worse by causing even more secretions to occur due to the stimulation. And most people find suctioning to be very uncomfortable. So usually, we don't.

"Also, you might see him begin to breathe faster. Sometimes, when we're close to dying, the body sends out signals that it's not getting enough oxygen. In response, the heart will begin to beat faster and the breathing rate will increase. If that happens, if he looks like he's beginning to labor a bit, elevate the head of the bed to forty-five degrees and prop his arms out a little, using pillows. This will keep his arms off his chest and open his chest a little more, making it easier for him to breathe. You can also place a fan nearby, on a low setting. Arrange it so the breeze is flowing across him, not directly at him. That will help."

"Would oxygen help, too?"

"Yes and no. It might help, but it can also cause discomfort."

"How so?"

"If he had a disease that prevented his lungs from functioning as they should, like cancer in his lungs, or emphysema, or COPD, then it would most likely help. But oxygen will also prolong his final hours. By interfering with his body's natural process, by asking his body to continue to function longer than it really can, we run the risk of causing other complications that wouldn't otherwise have occurred. So the first choice is to keep him comfortable just by repositioning him, using a fan or medications. But if this doesn't work, and he looks like he's working hard to breathe, call us.

"Also, a few people experience delirium, or agitation. But looking at Bob now, I don't think he will. He looks very peaceful. But if he does become agitated, call us.

"One other thing that's rare, but can be a problem, is jerking or twitching. Again, it's rare. But if it happens, call us. We'll want to change his medications to ensure that he stays comfortable.

"So if you see something that just doesn't feel right, like agitation, difficulty breathing, jerking, pain that isn't relieved by the medication, or any other concern, call us, day or night. We're here. We're here to support Bob and you and your whole family."

"Thank you," she whispers.

"You've noticed that the volume of urine has decreased, and that the urine looks fairly dark. Over time there'll be even less urine, and what he does put out will be very dark, more amber-colored. This tells us his kidneys are shutting down."

Bob's breathing pauses. Beverly turns to him and I watch as her head moves slightly, counting, marking off the seconds. Then Bob draws another breath. Beverly watches for a moment, then turns again to me.

"You saw me check his wrists and feet for pulses. Right now he has pulses at his wrists, and only faint pulses at his feet. As we move closer to dying, our circulation changes. Blood is drawn to our core. Because of this, his pulses will feel weak, or you may not be able to feel them at all. Also, his hands, feet, and knees will likely become cool, even cold. Right now, Bob's knees and feet are cool. When the extremities become cold, this can mean that the person is within several hours, or maybe less, of passing."

"Is that uncomfortable for him? Having cool feet and hands? Should I wrap them in a warm blanket?"

I shake my head. "Generally, people feel no discomfort from this change in circulation. In fact, when people this close to death are bundled up, often they'll attempt to remove what's covering them."

She nods and I continue. "If I were to take his blood pressure now, I'd find it to be low. Later I might not even be able to hear it. But I don't usually take blood pressure at this time. I can learn what I need to about how much longer he may be with us without disturbing him by squeezing his arm. At this time, I try to be as unobtrusive as possible."

Beverly smiles. "Thank you for that."

"Remember the discoloration I showed you on the sole of his right foot? That's called mottling. This is another response to the blood being drawn to our core. It's not uncomfortable in any way. Usually, the first places to mottle are the soles of the feet. You might also see mottling on his knees, his hands, and in later stages on his elbows or his thighs. Right now, Bob has very faint mottling. Sometimes, at least initially, mottling can come and go. But when it darkens to a deep, splotchy purple, and I see it in several places, I'll usually call the family to let them know their loved one might be within an hour or several hours of passing."

"So if I see that faint purple color becoming a lot darker, and occurring on more places, I should call the kids."

"Everyone is unique. It could mean he's very close, or it could be several hours or maybe even a day, and in some cases, longer. But if they want to be here, it would be a good idea to call them."

She glances at Bob, then turns to me and I continue. "I also look at facial coloring. Right now, Bob is a little pale, but there's still a natural tone to his face. When facial coloring becomes pallid, or ashen, that tells me a person may pass very soon, within moments, or maybe hours."

"So that's another change that would tell me to call the kids."

I nod. Then, in a quiet voice, I say, "The last change you'll see is a change in his breathing. It looks a lot like the way fish breathe when they're out of water. You'll see his lower jaw open fairly wide, then close.

He may take a few breaths like this. Those will be his last breaths."

She turns to Bob. Her thumb absently strokes the top of his hand as she holds it in hers. We sit together for some time. Neither of us speaks. I gaze at Beverly, at Bob, and silently wish them both a peaceful passage.

What a caterpillar calls the end of the world, the master calls a butterfly.
—Richard Bach

NEAR THE TIME OF DEATH
Observable Changes
You may see some or all of these changes as your loved one nears death:

- *A decreased level of consciousness* may occur within a week or two, to days before death. The person may be difficult to arouse, or may become completely unresponsive. Even if he's unresponsive, he may still be able to hear and be aware of who is present, what is said, and what is happening.
- Even if he's fully conscious, it's likely that he'll *take in no food or fluid* in the final days.
- *Incontinence of bladder and/or bowel* is likely to occur weeks to days prior to death.
- *Pauses in breathing,* lasting a few seconds to a minute or more, may occur weeks before death, though longer pauses may indicate that death will occur within days to hours.
- *Restlessness or disorientation* may occur in the weeks to days prior to death.
- *Talking with deceased loved ones and/or reaching for objects not seen by others* may occur weeks to days before death.
- *An inability to swallow* may occur several days prior to death.
- *Urine volume decreases, and urine becomes dark* in the last week to days.
- *A surge in energy* may occur in the days prior to death, resulting in the person being more alert and communicative.
- *Cooling hands, feet, and/or knees* may occur within days of death.
- Even as the extremities cool, *core body temperature may increase* in the final days.

- *Faint mottling of feet, knees, and/or hands* may occur within days prior to death; initially this may come and go.
- *Blood pressure may decrease; pulse and breathing rates may increase* in the days to hours before death.
- *Gurgling may be heard* from secretions at the back of the throat in the days to hours prior to death.
- *Cold hands, feet, and knees* usually indicate that death will occur within a day or two, or hours.
- *A weak or absent pulse at the wrists and/or feet* may indicate that death will occur within a day or two, or hours.
- *Skin coloring may become pallid* in the final few hours, or less.
- Significant *dark mottling of the feet, knees, hands, backs of the arms, and/or lower legs* usually signals that death will occur within hours, or sooner.
- *Jaw significantly lowers and closes with breaths:* These are the final breaths.
- *Absence of heartbeat and breathing, pupils enlarged:* The person has died.

When to Call Hospice

Call hospice if you see:

- Agitation or delirium unrelieved by medication
- Difficulty breathing, unrelieved by medication, repositioning, and use of fans
- Pain unrelieved by medication
- Jerking or twitching
- Other concerns

You should also call hospice at the time of death.

Additional Information

- For information on providing complete care, keeping your loved one comfortable, and giving necessary medications, see "How Do We Keep Her Comfortable?" (page 158).

- For information on using disposable underwear, see "How Do I Bring the Bathroom to Him?" (page 85).
- For information on creating a peaceful environment for your loved one, see "I Want to Be with Her When She Passes . . ." (page 179).
- For information on the experiences and awareness of people during the dying process, see "Will I Be Alone?" (page 6), "Will I Be Aware?" (page 13), and "Will I Choose My Time?" (page 9).
- For information on what to do at the time of death, see "I Want My Last Memory to Be a Good Memory . . ." (page 184).

I Want to Be With Her
🌺 When She Passes . . . 🌺

Meeting Your Loved One's Needs—
and Yours—in the Final Days
Ideas to Create a Peaceful Environment

Geraldine and Her Family

"WE'RE ALL HERE, JUST AS YOU ASKED us to be," says Roger, raising his voice to be heard as he leans toward his mother, Geraldine, as she lies unresponsive in a hospital bed in the center of the large living room.

I glance around the room at this impromptu family reunion, at the dozen or so young children playing on the floor, at the handful of teenagers slumped over noisy electronic games, at the adults: the men, alternately cheering and groaning at the sports game blaring from the TV, the women chatting and catching up with each other's lives. Then I gaze at Geraldine, in the center of it all. Her face appears relaxed, with the faint hint of a smile as her large, loving family gathers to share her last day or two.

Amidst this family gathering, the last "day or two" turns into several days, and still Geraldine lingers. Roger motions me out of the room and closes the French doors. "The doctor said she had a day or two, at most. We're here, just as she asked us to be. Why is she lingering?"

I glance through the glass doors and observe the noise and activity: the toys, the chatter, the TV. Through it all, Geraldine lies unresponsive, her face unchanged since the day her family arrived.

"Maybe she's just enjoying herself," Roger's sister Vivian says. "Maybe she's just so happy to have all of us here that she doesn't want to leave."

"Maybe . . . I don't know," Roger says. "She looks comfortable, but . . ." He runs a hand through his tousled hair. "What more can we do?"

"One thought might be to create a little more peaceful environment," I offer. "Another thought might be to give her some time alone."

Roger shakes his head. "The last time she was in the hospital, she told me that this is what she wanted, to have everyone with her when she died. So we're with her, day and night."

"And besides," Vivian adds. "I want to be with her when she passes. It's important to me."

I nod. "I've learned that, in the end, none of us really know what this moment will be like. We might believe that we'll want our loved ones with us, but when the moment arrives, it may be very different from what we thought it would be."

"Why do you think that?" Roger asks. "How can anyone know?"

"Let me tell you about a fellow named Chuck, and the lesson he taught us. Years ago I worked at a hospice where we believed no one should die alone. If a person didn't have loved ones or friends to be with him, we called volunteers who would sit quietly with the person until he or she passed. Day or night. Seven days a week. No one was left to die alone.

"One day we called volunteers to sit with this irascible but lovable man named Chuck, whom we believed would pass in the next twenty-four hours. Two weeks later we were still calling in volunteers. The doctors were amazed. We nurses were amazed. No one could understand how he could still be alive. But Chuck hung on. And so did the volunteers. Someone was always sitting beside Chuck, around the clock.

"Well, one day the volunteer who'd been sitting with Chuck approached me in the hall. His face was pale. His hands shook. 'I'm so sorry,' he uttered. 'I just stepped out for a moment. I had to go to the bathroom. When I came back . . .'

"It seems that Chuck took the first opportunity he'd had in more than two weeks to be alone, and had flown. We learned a lot from Chuck. After that, we still had volunteers to sit quietly with people, but the volunteers came and went, always offering the person some time alone, as well as a quiet, supportive presence."

Roger considers my words. Then he shakes his head. "She wanted us here."

"Whatever you feel is right for her. Though you might consider creating a quieter space," I add. "Sometimes, when we're close to passing, we don't like a lot of noise or stimulation, or even a lot of touch."

"How can you tell?" Vivian asks.

"Some people get restless. We consider that it might be pain, but we also consider the environment. Many times, when the environment calms down, so does the person. Once I was called to a home in the middle of the night. The woman was close to passing, but she was very restless. Like Geraldine, her large family had gathered to be with her. When I arrived, I found her family crowded in a circle around her bed, each of them stroking her arms and face and legs. This had gone on for hours: this constant touch, this circle of people around her bed.

"I asked them why they chose to do this, wondering if this was a cultural or religious tradition. But it wasn't. They said they just wanted to show her they were there, and that they loved her.

"We talked a bit, and finally they decided to step back and give her a little space. Within a few minutes, she settled down. Her restless arms stilled. Her breathing slowed. She remained peaceful for the next few hours, and then she took one long last breath and passed away."

"But Mom's not restless."

"She's made no response to any stimulation in over a week. She may not be physically able to show any sign of restlessness."

"Let's quiet things down a bit," Roger says, glancing back at the noisy room. "She might like that. But we're going to stay with her, just as she asked."

A few days later Roger again asks his question: "Why is she lingering?"

We talk in the hallway. "I'll talk to the rest of the family," he says. "See what they think, but I still don't think she's waiting to be alone."

Twenty minutes later he shares their answer. "We've decided to give her a little time alone. We've agreed to step out, but only for a little while. We'll come out here, to the hall. We'll give her fifteen minutes. Then we'll go back in."

My eyes widen at such a short amount of time, but this is their choice. "How can I support your family?" I ask.

Roger shrugs. "I don't know. Just wait with us, maybe."

One by one, family members file past Geraldine's bed. Each bends close to kiss her cheek, then whispers some reassurance in her ear, "We'll be just outside the door. We're going to step out for fifteen minutes. Then we'll be right back in." Through it all Geraldine's face remains unchanged.

After the last family member approaches the bed, we all begin to file out the door. As I turn to close the French doors behind us, I hear Geraldine's breathing change. I hesitate, listening, watching as her jaw begins that deep lowering and closing motion, the last breaths. Silently, I wish her a peaceful journey, and close the doors.

Without mysteries, life would be very dull indeed. What would be left to strive for if everything were known?

— Charles de Lint

IDEAS FOR CREATING AND SHARING A PEACEFUL ENVIRONMENT

At this time, many people prefer a quiet environment with minimal stimulation. To create and share this space, consider the following approaches:

* Sit quietly in the room, using this time for silent reflection or to say good-bye.
* Set aside time alone for your loved one. When you're preparing to leave, say good-bye, and tell her when you'll return. Accept that this may be the last time you see her.
* Accept that your loved one may choose the time that's right for her to pass.
* Consider that your loved one may be aware of and able to hear what is said nearby.

- When touching your loved one, consider passively holding her hand or offer a very light touch, as opposed to a more active, stroking touch.
- Cover your loved one only with a sheet or a light blanket. Oftentimes, people nearing death don't want to be covered with heavy blankets.
- If religious practice is an important part of your loved one's life, discuss with her spiritual leader what prayers, recitations, or other offerings might be appropriate at this time.
- Allow pets to be present.
- If your loved one enjoys music, consider low-volume, soothing music.
- If your loved one enjoys being outdoors, consider moving the bed outside in good weather. Provide shade if the sun is bright. Monitor her temperature if the weather is hot or cold.
- Avoid bright, artificial lighting in the room. In the evening and at night, use low lighting when needed.
- Avoid strong fragrances, such as heavily scented candles, heavy perfumes, and certain flowers.
- Most important, be at peace, and share this peace with your loved one.
- For more information about signs of approaching death, see "How Will We Know When the End Is Near?" (page 170).

I Want My Last Memory
to Be a Good Memory . . .

What to Do at the Time of Death
Ideas for Honoring and Caring for Your
Loved One at the Time of Death

Peter and Lauren

"So . . . when the time comes, do we call you?" Peter asks, reaching for his sister Lauren's hand as we sit together at their mother's kitchen table.

"Yes, when she passes you call hospice. If you would like, someone from hospice can come to your home, day or night, to support your family, but that's up to you. There are a number of other things you can also do, depending on what's right for your family.

"In hospice, we honor the person in life and at her passing. How each family honors their loved one is up to them. Some families find it helpful to follow the traditions of their faith. Some gather at the bedside to share stories of how their loved one enriched their lives. Some choose not to be present at all. There's no one right approach.

"For many families though, having some kind of observance immediately after the death is helpful. Instead of leaving the room, closing the door, and waiting for the funeral home representative to arrive, families may be able to transform this time from one of loss, from the image of the lifeless body, to a time of a remembrance, an honoring of their loved one."

"How do they do that?" Lauren asks.

"At the time of death, the first thing many do is simply sit with their loved one. No matter how prepared we think we are, none of us know what we'll feel at that time. We need time just to take it in.

"When they're ready, some families choose to bathe the body. For some, this cleansing is part of their religious tradition; for others, it's simply an act of love. After the bathing, they comb the hair and dress their loved one in something loose and easy to slip on. Some families ask friends to help; others ask hospice; some choose to involve only close family. And some families choose not to do this at all. Again, it's up to each family—what's right for them.

"Some traditions call for a ceremonial covering to be placed over the person. It may be a simple white sheet, a woven blanket, or a quilt, depending on the tradition. In most cases, the covering is arranged to leave the person's face uncovered. The arms are laid atop the cover. Sometimes a flower or another item with special meaning is placed in the loved one's hands.

"At this time some families choose to offer a prayer or a reading, depending on their faith or traditions. Some choose to share stories about their loved one, their favorite memories, or funny stories. I've been privileged to be part of many of these gatherings. What I find most remarkable is how the essence of the person really comes through in these stories."

"How so?" Peter asks.

"Well, a few nights ago, I shared this time with another family. The woman's children, all grown adults with their own children, gathered immediately after her passing. According to her spiritual traditions, we bathed her, then dressed her in a gown of her favorite colors. We then placed a special quilt over her, leaving her face uncovered. Her children lit a candle. Then they each read a passage from the Kaddish. Afterward, they began to share their favorite memories. In these stories, without any planning or forethought, a theme began to emerge of how she had an uncanny way of knowing when she was needed, even as they grew older. They shared story after story of how she could astound and surprise them with just the right action, even though she couldn't possibly have known the circumstances that preceded her actions.

"After they shared memories, they opened a bottle of sparkling cider, pouring each person a glass, as well as a glass for her. Then they raised their glasses to all that she had taught them, by example, about leading a meaningful life, and to the extraordinary spirit she was, and still is within each of them.

"When the funeral home representative arrived, they asked the gentleman to leave the passage quilt over her, with her face uncovered, for her journey from her home to his van. Some of her children chose to accompany her out. Some did not. Each chose what they wanted to carry in their memories."

Lauren reaches for a tissue and wipes her eyes. "Whatever we do, I want my last memory to be a good memory."

In the Native way we are encouraged to recognize that every moment is a sacred moment, and every action, when imbued with dedication and commitment to benefit all beings, is a sacred act.

—*Dhyani Ywahoo*

At the Time of Death

Observances to Consider

For more information about customs and traditions of your faith, consult your spiritual leader.

You may also consider other observances, including:

- Bathing, dressing, and grooming the body
- Cutting a lock of hair
- Lighting a candle at the bedside
- Placing a quilt or coverlet over your loved one, leaving the face exposed
- Sharing stories and favorite or funny memories
- Offering a toast

Calling Hospice at the Time of Death

After your loved one has died, take the time you need. Then, when you are ready, call hospice. The hospice nurse will ask the following questions:

- What time did your loved one pass?
- Would you like someone from hospice to come to your location to support you? (Some hospices automatically make a visit at the time

of death. If you don't want them to visit, you may decline, unless a visit is required by local law.)

- How are you and others who are with you coping?
- Are you ready for the funeral home representative to be called to come to your location? (If you are going to observe traditions or gather at the bedside to share stories, ask hospice to call the funeral home after this is completed.)

When you're ready, hospice will call the funeral home and request that a representative come to your location.

After your loved one has died, if a hospice nurse doesn't visit, you will be instructed on how to dispose of unused medications. By law you will be required to dispose of certain medications. For information about donating usable medications and supplies to international medical relief agencies, visit this guide's Web site for current information: www.LivingAtTheEndofLife.com

What Hospice Does Following a Death

- Hospice notifies the person's doctor, the medical examiner, the pharmacy, the remaining hospice staff, and the hospice volunteer(s) involved in supporting your family.
- Hospice arranges for all medical equipment to be picked up from your location.
- A hospice representative will contact you with information about grief support.

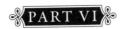

❧ PART VI ❧

How Will I Go On? Coping with Loss

This section offers information that may be helpful to loved ones beginning their grieving process.

This section provides an introduction to the journey of grief, an ever-changing process that each of us experiences in our own way. You'll learn about common physical and emotional changes you may experience, as well as tools and resources to help you understand and cope.

I Feel So Alone . . .
An Introduction to Grief and Bereavement

How Are You?
How Love and Loss Shape Who We Are

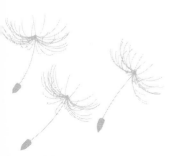

❀ I Feel So Alone ... ❀

An Introduction to Grief and Bereavement

Len

"Thank you," I say, accepting the quilt, spreading it in my arms to admire the artful blending of colors and theme, lovingly stitched together.

"The ladies at my church made it. I told them about the tradition of passage quilts, and they wanted to make one for the hospice in her honor," says Len, whose wife Jean passed away here at the hospice house two months before.

"Thank you. It's beautiful."

Len nods. His eyes mist.

"How are you?" I ask.

He shrugs. "I get by."

"You look a bit thinner than I recall."

"Not much of an appetite." With one finger he traces the outline of a wild iris in the quilt, then adds. "I wasn't sure I could come here today." He gazes around the room. "A lot of memories here." He tries to smile. "Some days it feels good to be around the things she loved. Other days I go out of my way to avoid anything that will remind me of her." He exhales a long, slow breath. "I dream about her. They're wonderful dreams. But then I wake up and I feel so alone." He leans toward me. I gather him in my arms with the quilt pressed between us.

"I think that's the hardest part ... these swings," he whispers into my shoulder. "One day I think I'm making progress, the next it's as if I can't do anything but cry." He draws back. "I'm not going to do this," he says, wiping his tears. "I promised myself this would be a happy occasion, coming here, thanking all of you, giving you this quilt."

"I suspect most happy occasions still have their sadness."

"Should I be feeling like this? One minute happy, the next, ready to break down and cry? And sometimes, when I *am* happy, I feel guilty."

I lead him to an alcove and we settle on the window seat. "As strange as it seems, yes, that's actually quite common. A lot of things that don't feel 'normal' actually are."

"Like what?"

"Like coming here, where you can be with people who understand your loss. People who grieve often choose to spend time with close friends, people with whom they can share their story. At the same time, while people who grieve respond to kindness and warmth, they also appreciate being left alone. Just knowing they can turn to their friends is comforting.

"And feeling happy, then feeling guilty about being happy, is common, too. So are mood swings: feeling happy or sad, or angry, or any number of other emotions—all within a short period—and not being able to pinpoint why, or what triggered the change of emotion."

"That's one of the harder things to deal with. My friends have really been wonderful, inviting me to dinner, or lunch. Sometimes we'll all be having a nice evening and suddenly I'll just want to cry, or be alone . . . You'd think I could control it, but it just comes over me, for no apparent reason." Len sighs. "How long will that last?"

"Everyone has their own time line. Eventually, you'll probably have these episodes less frequently. Or you might go for a while without one, then suddenly, after days, weeks, or months even, feel it again. But over time, this overwhelming sadness will pass. Eventually, you'll be able to think of her, to recall your time together and feel happiness without also feeling the powerful sense of loss you feel now. But if these frequent, strong swings of emotion do continue more than another few months, you might consider some additional grief support."

"I got the information hospice sent on support groups, and I talked to the social worker. I thought that when Jean died, hospice was finished, but . . . Thanks for still being here for me. If I feel I need it, I'll take you up on that." He reaches for my hand. "What else can I expect to feel?"

"People who grieve often have physical responses. You mentioned that you have vivid dreams. That's common. You also mentioned a decrease in appetite. That's common, too. It's also common for people to eat far more than they used to and gain weight. Some people channel their grief through exercise. Some people—even those who have been very physically active—become sedentary. A lot of people experience difficulty sleeping, and wake up tired. People's physical responses vary."

"Throughout the day I can keep busy, or at least think that I'm busy. Mostly I just flit from one thing to another, not really getting anything done. But at least I'm doing something. At night . . . at night, I lie there, and there's nothing to distract me, nothing but the emptiness . . . I just lie there, for hours sometimes. It's the hollowness, just this cold, empty feeling. For so long she was there, beside me. I felt her warmth. I heard her breathe. And now . . . Now I'm alone."

His gaze wanders out the window to the garden. "I haven't been much of a religious man, but I find myself thinking about a higher being, that maybe there's some purpose to all of this." He turns to me. "Do you have any answers for that?"

I offer a rueful smile. "I'm afraid not. That's something each of us has to figure out, in our own way."

Absently he fingers the quilt, tracing the outlines of flowers, leaves, earth, water, sky. He closes his eyes. "I miss her."

The pain passes, but the beauty remains.

—Pierre-Auguste Renoir

Grief Work
By Patrick L. Clary

Weeks after the funeral
Only one pair of sparrows
Puzzled over dooryard snow
Blank after sixty years of crumbs.

I was done talking,
Done feeding those flocks of birds with him *gone,*
Done tolerating a kitchen full of visitors
Expressing sympathy for the loss
I thought of as desertion:
Next stop—nursing home.

That pretty hospice volunteer mixed
Warm water, yeast and flour before
I threw her *out—*
But I kept the fragrant dough
She left rising beside the woodstove,
To knead, and slash, and beat it
Gray as stones—
Unfit for human consumption.

Over-salted as it was
By sweat and tears,
I baked it anyway.

Too hard to cut,
The flat loaf shatters
Under my husband's hammer,
I pound shards to dusty chunks
Sweep it all up in my apron,
And scatter the whole mess
Into the swirl
Of all those returning, vigilant birds.

Patrick L. Clary, *Dying for Beginners*, Lost Borders Press

COMMON GRIEF EXPERIENCES AND RESOURCE INFORMATION

Styles of Grief

Grief is a uniquely personal experience, shaped by many factors, among them:

+ Your relationship with the person who died
+ The circumstances of the death
+ Your personality style
+ Your support system
+ Your cultural practices
+ Your spiritual practices
+ Your religious traditions

These factors influence how you will express and cope with your grief. Even within the same family, expressions of grief may differ significantly. Some people might be more vocal and expressive in their grief, while others may quietly contemplate or channel their feelings into activities. Because of these differences, tensions can arise within families that have experienced loss. Recognize that while the expressions of grief and ways of coping may differ among individuals, each person feels the pain of the loss.

For many of us, family provides our greatest source of support. In situations where everyone within the family is grieving, seek other sources of support for yourself, and encourage other family members to do the same, in a way that's right for them.

Support comes in many forms, among them friends, spirituality, activities, support groups, and books. Keep in mind that a form of support that one person finds very helpful, might not be right for you, or right for you at that time. Consider exploring different resources. Just as different books have different styles and messages, grief support groups can also vary widely in the dynamics of the group. If the resource you've chosen doesn't feel right for you, consider trying a different group, book, or other tool.

Hospice Support Resources

U.S. Medicare–certified hospice programs offer grief support to anyone in their community who has experienced a loss, even if they did not participate in hospice prior to the loss. Many offer support groups, guided by a grief counselor. Some also offer support to meet the special needs of children experiencing grief, before and after the loss. Contact your local hospice for more information.

Grief Books

While you might find it helpful to have a "Ten Best Grief Books" list, most bereavement counselors agree that no such list exists. The way people feel and express grief varies widely. Consequently, the way people cope and evolve with their grief varies widely, too.

The best approach to locating a book that meets your particular style and needs would be to visit your local bookstore or library and spend some time exploring different books. Read the first few pages. Then skip ahead to a later chapter and read a few pages there. How do you feel about what you've read? Can you see yourself in those passages? Can you see yourself taking the actions the author recommends, and finding comfort in these actions? Take your time. Explore a few books. Take a break. Maybe wander different aisles, or just sit quietly. When you're ready, go back and explore another book or two. And if nothing feels right, give yourself permission to leave this task unfinished and come back another day. Remember that grief takes a physical and mental toll on each of us. Everything: decision making, getting up in the morning, falling asleep . . . it all takes more time than it used to. Give yourself that time. You are healing, and that, too, takes time.

Common Physical Responses to Grief

- A feeling of tightness in the chest or throat, or the feeling of a "pit" in your stomach
- A change in appetite, either an increase or decrease
- A change in physical activity, including feelings of lethargy, or a desire to exercise frequently
- Periods of frequent crying or sighing
- Difficulty falling asleep or remaining asleep

Common Emotional or Cognitive Responses to Grief

- When you're awake, your loss may be present in most of your thoughts. Over time, this preoccupation will likely decrease; you will be able to think about other things, and thoughts of your loss will occur less frequently.

- When you're asleep, you may experience vivid dreams about your loved one and the loss.

- You may find your mood changing frequently, with more extremes of emotion than you usually experience.

- You may experience sudden feelings of sadness, even when participating in enjoyable activities.

- You may feel guilty about experiencing enjoyment in life.

- You may feel a need to stay busy.

- You may seek the company of close friends and want to talk with them about your feelings.

- You may find sitting with others and talking about your loss (such as in a support group) to be helpful.

- You may find comfort in creating objects, such as photo collages or other memorials.

- You may seek time to be alone, but appreciate knowing you can call on friends or loved ones for support when you want to talk or be near others.

- Your ability to concentrate may be diminished. Consequently, you may feel overwhelmed or frustrated performing even simple tasks or handling decision making.

- You may think about what your loved one would want you to do, but feel guilty that you aren't able to do it.

- You may spend more time exploring your spiritual beliefs, and may question previously held beliefs.

❀ HOW ARE YOU? ❀

How Love and Loss Shape Who We Are

"I TOOK CARE OF MY FATHER. I WAS WITH him when he died . . ."

Instantly, I become still. My posture changes, opens. It is time to listen.

The man's eyes moisten with tears. "Boy, I don't know what's gotten into me. It's been years since Dad died . . ."

I am not working. I'm not in a family's home or kneeling beside a hospital bed. I'm at a gas station. As I'd lowered the window to ask the attendant for a fill-up, he noticed my work badge: *Karen B., Hospice RN.*

For many of us, telling our story is part of healing. Soon after a death, our loved ones, friends, and community support us in our grief. They listen as we share our stories. They bring food. They sit patiently as we cry.

But that support may not last as long as we need it to. We live in a culture that isn't always comfortable with intimacy. And grief—with all its emotional pain—can be searingly intimate. In our culture we ask, "How's the weather?" far more easily than we ask, "How are you?" So after a while we stop sharing our stories. We stop reaching out. We close off what we feel. We go on with our lives.

But I Should Be Over This . . .

When people discover what I do for a living, memories that have long since been stored away, like photos in a box that's been carried to the basement, rush to the surface, the emotions as vivid and raw as if the loss had occurred only recently. Tearfully, they share their stories—at gas stations, at dinner parties, in grocery store parking lots—surprised and sometimes embarrassed by what they have shared, by what they feel. "But I should be over this," they say, disconcerted, looking away, as if feeling in the dark to find again a safe and familiar place.

When Will Things Feel "Normal" Again?

"Normal" is the life we knew with our loved one. Life after our loss will be different. For a time it will be painful. That focus that has consumed us—caring for and being with our loved one—abruptly ends. And if we've been a caregiver for a long period, we may feel a loss not only for the one we love, but also for the role we played—giving care, giving of ourselves, our moments filled with fulfilling their needs.

But after their passing, we must deal with our own needs. And for that there are no easy answers. Grief creates conflict within us. An important element of our lives is irrevocably changed. We cannot go back to what once was. We can only go forward. And often, we don't know how. How *do* we resolve this pain, this imbalance, this emptiness we feel?

Each of us will find the way that's right for us. We might talk about it. We might find tasks to stay busy, to channel our restless energy. We might turn to books to help us cope. We might attend grief groups. We might take long walks.

One day we take the box of photos to the basement. "That's done," we say. Our fingers linger, just for a moment, on the lifeless cardboard edges. Then we climb the stairs, switch off the light, and close the door. That's done.

Or is it?

How Long Does Grief Last?

In truth, some part of that feeling of loss remains with us. It always will. But so, too, remains the essence of the life and love we shared, perhaps in more ways then we realize. In sharing life with someone, in sharing love, we can, perhaps, become wiser, stronger, kinder, better able to give, better able to reach out to another, better able to be patient, better able to forgive.

In living and loving, in feeling the happiness as well as the loss and pain, we are better able to stand amidst strangers and realize that we are not strangers. We are forever connected, the past and the present, our hopes and needs, one living being to another.

I stand beside the man as he pumps the gas. "How are you?" I ask.

What we have once enjoyed we can never lose . . .
All that we love deeply becomes a part of us.

—Helen Keller

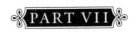

❧ PART VII ❧

Living

This section offers information that may be helpful to anyone affected by loss, and can be read at any time during this journey.

This section relates some of the remarkable lessons I've been offered about life and living from individuals and families who have shared their journey with me. I share their courage, grace, and wisdom with you, in hopes that you, too, will discover your own path to meaning, hope, and peace.

Is There Life after Death?
Does It Influence How I Live Now?

Can I Choose How I Live?

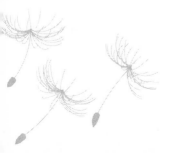

❈ Is There Life After Death? ❈

Does It Influence How I Live Now?

WHAT BEGINS AFTER THE LAST BREATH IS let go? When our heart no longer beats? What begins when what we know and understand ends? What becomes of our soul?

Many years ago, when I first began practice as a hospice nurse, I was asked this question: Is there life after death? Then, as now, I have no answer. I do not know. Perhaps someday I will know, when I, too, let go that last breath, when I, too, make this journey.

For now, what I've come to understand is that we live among people who understand, not what will be after the last breath, but what can be with this breath, this life, this moment. They live with a clarity of purpose, with compassion, kindness, and grace. From them I've learned not to ask, "What will be?" but rather, "What is now?" From them I've learned that it's possible to live that afterlife—that paradise, that heaven, that rebirth—to forge a better existence, now.

Billy

I met Billy in New Orleans, where I served as a volunteer shortly after Hurricanes Katrina and Rita devastated the region. Billy volunteered in the "Yard," and became known as the "Yard Dog." Every morning, just after dawn, hundreds of volunteers like me converged on the vast grounds of the church that hosted a coalition of the American Red Cross and the Southern Baptist Convention, with their cargo containers, refrigerator trucks, portable kitchens, and a fleet of Emergency Response Vehicles (ERVs) to deliver disaster relief.

Billy was the first to arrive each morning, in the predawn hours, and he was one of the last to leave. He held no official title or rank, and it was he who dubbed himself the "Yard Dog." Working at a brisk pace, bordering on a run, he loaded pallets with water bottles, juices, hot meal containers, utensil packages, and the countless other supplies needed to feed and respond to the needs of thousands of families as they attempted to reclaim their homes and restart their lives.

By the time the rest of us came on the scene, Billy and a small crew had managed to place a full day's supply behind each of our twenty-three ERVs. All we needed to do was load and secure the supplies, attend the day's briefing, and then depart on our routes.

While we delivered meals, attended to cuts and scrapes, and brightened lives that had been devastated by natural disaster, Billy prepared for the next day, unloading semis and organizing supplies beneath enormous, circus-sized white tents, always at that same rapid pace, never tiring, never faltering.

When we returned at dusk, he was there to greet us, to lend a strong hand, an encouraging voice, words of thanks for our efforts, when, in truth, he had done far more than we ever had. For our efforts, we witnessed the smiles and garnered the appreciation of those we had come to serve as we offered a hot meal and a cold drink. Billy, who rarely left the yard, saw none of that. For him the reward was sending us on our way, fully loaded, prepared and able to give, and give more.

At the end of the day, each ERV team was required to wash its ERV's meal containers—Cambros, as we called them, for the brand name stamped prominently on the side. Cleaning Cambros required first disposing of the unused food, which by this hour had become cold and greasy. We then rinsed the container—a job that required considerable skill with a hose, lest we splash cold, congealed ground beef or macaroni and cheese all over ourselves. After a good rinsing, the Cambro moved down the line, through the wash, through the sanitizer, and finally to the dry line. It was a job almost everyone avoided, or grumbled about when it couldn't be avoided. But for Billy, it was the highlight of the day. "The Zen of Cambro," he called it: doing the job no one else wanted to do; serving with joy, with laughter, with purpose.

He taught me that Zen. And he taught others. Over the course of my stay, many still avoided Cambro cleaning, and made no secret of their distaste for that chore. But others sought it out, playfully bumping each other from the line for our turn with the rinse hose or the soapy water, only to be bumped again, moments later. Amidst the spray of water, laughter echoed and friends were made. We came together from many different walks of life, different ages, different religions, and different cultures, united by our sense of purpose, and the joy of helping others.

One morning, late in my stay, Billy came to say good-bye. He returned to his home and his family, and another volunteer stepped in and tried to fill the enormous shoes of the "Yard Dog."

Is there life after death? I don't know. But I have to ask: In living life, in choosing how we interact with our fellow living beings and with our home—the planet—does it matter? Is the reward for a life of kindness heaven, or paradise, or rebirth to a better existence? Is our giving contingent on this reward? Or are we content to be rewarded simply by giving, with what may come to remain a mystery, to be known only when that moment arrives?

Whatever our faith, whatever its teachings, at their core, whether Christian, Muslim, Hindu, Jewish, Buddhist, Native American, another Native tradition, or any other of this world's many views of life, all hold a single guiding principle: compassion for our fellow living beings and the world we share.

What has our life been? What is it now? What light lives within our soul? How brightly do we let it shine?

There are two ways to live your life: One is as if nothing is a miracle, and the other is as if everything is a miracle.

—Albert Einstein

THE JOURNEY AT THE END OF LIFE IS, IN TRUTH, a continuation of the journey of life. Here, all that we did, all that we did not do, the values we hold, what we believe in, are brought sharply into focus. We experience fears, courage, doubts, anger, love, grief, sadness, redemption, and hope. We wonder, "Am I living, or am I dying?"

In these moments, yes, a part of us is dying. We are limited by our failing bodies. We are saying good-bye. We are grieving. We are preparing for the end of what we know.

But in these moments we are also living. With each breath we still possess the capacity to choose—not what happens to us in life, but how we respond. Collectively, these choices shape our lives. The outcomes of these choices are what we look back on when the end draws near, what we are remembered for, what we leave behind, and, perhaps, what we take with us as we leave. In these remaining months, weeks, days, hours, we are living. We can still choose how we live.

I witness this every day among those whose bodies are failing, and those who will soon be without the one they love. Amidst the struggle of dying, they live.

Mona

"We waited for you," she says, standing outside the doors of the hospice house as I arrive. Visible in the fragile light of early dawn, her face shows weariness, and the release that came finally, late in the night. "I didn't want them to come for him without you having a chance to say good-bye."

For a moment we stand together, each silently acknowledging the journey we have shared. Two months earlier, Mona arrived at the hospice, suitcase in hand. She'd driven most of the day from the small farming community where she'd been raised, where she raised her own family, attended church potlucks, and helped her neighbors during calving season and harvest. Arriving at the hospice, her face showed the determination of the farmwife she was—an expectation that things would be difficult, but an unshakable belief that this tilling of the soil, this nursing of a dying son, was the greatest purpose life could offer.

Years before, she'd cut off all ties with him. In the eyes of her faith, he lived an immoral life. She sided with her faith. He got on with his life. He contributed to society, achieved professional success, and, one day, while traveling on business in Singapore, he collapsed.

And so the mother who had cast out her son packed a single suitcase, slid behind the wheel of her Plymouth, and drove west, past her church, past the rolling farmlands, past the differences in beliefs, the hurtful words, the years of silence, and arrived at his door.

Later we learned just how much that had cost her. The church shunned her. Her family hurled angry words at her. But still she came.

And she stayed—through the weakness, the confusion, the diarrhea, the seizures, the fear, the hope, the reconciliation, and, finally, the peace, found in a mother's arms. Once again, she became his mother. And she became mother to all the other motherless, abandoned boys who came through our doors in those early days of AIDS. She welcomed them into her ample arms and cradled them with a love that understands and accepts that life, at times, can be cruel and unfair. But still, it is life. And in those last months of her son's life, in those months of her life, she had a choice about how she would live.

Eventually, she returned to her community where she once again attended church potlucks and helped neighbors during calving season and harvest. Among her neighbors, any unkind words or uncharitable thoughts were checked before they could be fully formed. For, in the character of her face, in the sureness of her hands, there was a quiet conviction, an unshakable strength borne from loving and losing a son, from a realization that life is full of birth and death, of happiness and the need for courage. It is life. It is living.

"We waited for you," she says. We take each other's hand and go inside.

Sunny

She was a secretary by day, and a soulful jazz singer by night. Raised in a strict Jewish household, Sunny, at the youthful bloom of fifty-four, broke free of the traditions and expectations that defined her life and joined the Lakota Sioux Indian tribe. There she learned their spiritual practices and beliefs, and incorporated these into her life.

I met her ten years later, when cancer claimed much of her vibrant energy and left her, at times, confused. And yet there was something remarkable about her, something deep and wise and insightful that defied the disease, the limitations, the impermanence of the mere physical human form.

Since the early days of writing this guide, I have wondered how to share her spirit. But a life, and the wisdom of a lifetime, cannot be captured in a few paragraphs. A lifetime is just that—a lifetime. It is joy, heartache, growth, happiness. It is challenge, fear, love, hope. She lived them all, with a sparkle in her eyes, with tenacity, with exasperation, with compassion and generosity. She made mistakes. She touched lives.

She was never rich, and most of the time she struggled to make ends meet. But this never bothered her. "What's life without a little challenge?" she would say with a shrug. "That's how you learn, you know."

I wonder what she would say, this wise, funny lady, if she knew that one day I would look back to the time we shared for the right words to say to those who follow her in this journey, your journey, and someday mine, too.

I think she would tell me there is no guide. There are practical tips, insights, and caring words of support—all helpful, all needed. But for the things that matter most, there is only love, and hope, and these alone will guide you.

To those who shake their heads and say, "What is there to hope for?" I imagine she would smile that crooked smile of hers, chuckle, and reply, "Ah, there's so much . . . so much to hope for. If you only knew . . ."

She knew. She knew something most of us can only wonder about. How else can it be explained that this frumpy lady who ambled about in worn slippers and baggy sweatpants, who often didn't know what day it was, or what happened yesterday, could walk up to people, look into their eyes, and read their soul?

This happened not once, but often. Many mornings as I arrived at the hospice, she would shuffle up to me, first with a look of puzzlement, then dawning recognition. She would place her hands on my shoulders, look into my eyes, and proceed to offer advice on the very problem that was troubling me, though she could not possibly have known.

And now, finally, I think I understand the wisdom she couldn't put into words, but could only show me. To understand, I had to travel this journey, all the years, all the families, all their journeys of hope and healing, release and rebirth.

In the big picture of life, does it really matter what day it is, or what happened yesterday? Could it be that what's most important is this moment, right now? This moment, the moment we live now.

What will you do with the life you have left?

Will you live any differently?

As you take your final breaths, will you be at peace?

Do you know why you live?

I wanted a perfect ending. Now I've learned, the hard way, that some poems don't rhyme, and some stories don't have a clear beginning, middle, and end. Life is about not knowing. It's about having to change, taking the moment and making the best of it, without knowing what's going to happen next.

—Gilda Radner

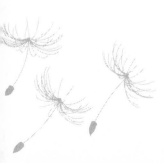

To finish the moment, to find the journey's end in every step of the road, to live the greatest number of good hours, is wisdom.

—Ralph Waldo Emerson

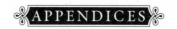

❧ APPENDIX A ❧
Additional Resources

For updated information and Web site links, visit this guide's Web site, www.LivingAtTheEndOfLife.com

General Resource Support

To learn more about a variety of end-of-life topics, visit www.HospiceNet.org.

For U.S. Residents: To access a variety of tools and information about end-of-life issues, visit the Web site of the National Hospice & Palliative Care Organization, www.CaringInfo.org.

For assistance in locating services and financial resources in your area, visit www.Eldercare.gov, or call Eldercare Locator at 1-800-677-1116, to be directed to the nearest office of the Area Agency on Aging.

For UK Residents: To locate information about resources available to UK residents, visit the Web site of Help the Hospices, www.helpthehospices.org.uk, keywords *About Hospice Care.*

For Canadian Residents: To locate information about resources available to Canadian residents, visit the Web site of the Canadian Hospice & Palliative Care Association, www.CHPCA.net.

For Residents of All Other Countries: To locate hospice resources available in other countries, visit the Web site of Help the Hospices, www.helpthehospices.org.uk, keyword *International.*

Medical Decision Making

For more information about treatment choices, such as resuscitation (CPR), artificial feeding, or other life support, read *Hard Choices for Loving People,* by Hank Dunn. This short, compassionately written booklet helps families better understand these complex issues. The booklet is available at www.HardChoices.com.

For U.S. Residents: For free, downloadable Advance Directive and Medical Power of Attorney forms for every U.S. state and the District of Columbia, visit www.CaringInfo.org, keywords *Planning Ahead,* or call the helpline at 1-800-658-8898.

Caregiving Support

To learn more about caregiving resources and to download helpful, free publications, visit the Web site for the National Alliance for Caregiving, www.Caregiving.org. This site also offers the Family Care Resource Connection to help you select instructional materials to meet your specific caregiving needs.

Other good sources of information about caregiving include the Family Caregiver Alliance, www.Caregiver.org, and Help the Hospices, www.helpthehospices.org.uk, keywords *Help and Support for Carers.*

Financial Support

For U.S. Residents: To determine what financial assistance you may be eligible for, visit www.AARP.org. Locate the *Benefits QuickLINK* resource on the site. *Benefits QuickLINK* helps you find and enroll in public and private benefits programs available for older adults and families with children. You can use the site's Application Forms Center to print out an application or apply online. Other useful information is also available at this site.

You can also locate this information at www.BenefitsCheckUp.org. This site offers similar search tools to locate public and private assistance for which you may be eligible.

You can also contact your county's Office of Aging Services to learn what services or resources are available in your community.

For UK Residents: To locate information about financial support, visit Help the Hospices at www.helpthehospices.org.uk, keywords *Financial Benefits for Carers.*

Volunteer Support

To help organize the support of your friends and loved ones, visit www. LotsaHelpingHands.com, a free Internet service that allows you to set up a secure, online list of activities (i.e., meal making, errand running, etc.) that your supporters can view and sign up for. This site also allows you to securely post updates for your support network.

Communication Tools

To securely post updates that designated people (loved ones, friends, etc.) can view, visit www.LotsaHelpingHands.com or www.CaringBridge. org. Both offer free, secure Internet posting services.

To access free, Internet-based audio and video communication services, visit www.Skype.com.

For more information about sending large digital files (including digital video clips) via the Internet, visit www.YouSendIt.com.

Selecting a Care Facility, Determining Costs, Paying for Care

For U.S. Residents: To locate information about long-term care facilities in your area, visit www.Medicare.gov, keywords *Nursing Home Compare.* This tool provides quality ratings, checklists, and tips on how to select the right care facility for you. This site does not provide information about adult foster homes.

Another good source of information about locating and paying for care facilities or in-home private care is www.AARP.org, keywords *Long Term Care.* Here you'll find a variety of tools for evaluating paid caregiving options, determining approximate costs, and other useful information. This site provides limited information about adult foster homes.

To determine if you are eligible for Medicaid or Supplemental Security Income benefits for paid caregiving, talk with a social worker or visit www.AARP.org, keywords *Benefits QuickLINK* (see Financial Support above). Fill out the online questionnaire to determine eligibility.

To locate and research adult foster homes in your community, talk with a social worker. In the United States, information about adult foster homes may be available through your state's Department of Health and Human Services.

For Canadian Residents: Visit www.CHPCA.net and search for resources by province or territory.

Accessing Palliative Care

Palliative care is similar to hospice in that it focuses on relief of pain and other symptoms of serious illness. Both strive to prevent or ease suffering, and to facilitate the best possible quality of life. Unlike hospice, palliative care is appropriate at any stage of a serious illness and is not dependent on life expectancy. It can be provided at the same time as curative or life-prolonging treatment. To learn more about palliative care, visit www. GetPalliativeCare.org or www.PalliativeDoctors.org.

Associations Offering Resources or Information

American Cancer Society: www.cancer.org

American Heart Association: www.americanheart.org

American Lung Association: www.lungusa.org

Alzheimer's Association: www.alz.org

National Kidney Foundation: www.kidney.org

The ALS Association: www.alsa.org

Macmillan Cancer Support: www.cancerlink.org (UK resource)

Other disease-specific associations may also offer information and resources.

Purchasing Medical Equipment

Should you need medical equipment not provided by hospice, consider visiting www.craigslist.org, a free classified ad service that allows you to search for needed items for sale in your community. Items offered through this site are generally used, and are often priced well below the retail price if you were to buy them new.

Estate Planning (Wills)

For large or complex estate planning, consult an attorney. For less complex estate planning, consider *Quicken WillMaker Plus Estate Planning Essentials*, a book packaged with a CD. This resource walks you through preparing a legally binding will and other important legal documents.

Donating Unused Medications and Medical Supplies

Some medications and supplies can be donated to medical relief agencies. For current information about what can be donated and where to send these items, visit this guide's Web site, www.LivingAtTheEndOfLife.com

Grief Support

To locate grief support groups in your community, contact your local hospice.

To find the right resource book for you, visit your local bookstore or library. Plan to spend some time exploring the style and contents of different books to select the right one for you.

If you are considering adopting a pet, please consider adopting from a shelter or rescue organization, where pets—cats, dogs, and other domestic animals—are available in all sizes and breeds, from mixed breeds to purebreds. Each year in the United States, more than seven million animals become homeless. Many are euthanized. In making this choice, you will literally be saving a loving animal's life.

To learn more about pet adoption or to locate an animal seeking a new, loving home in your community, visit the free search service www.PetFinder. com. Simply enter your zip code and preferences (dog, cat, size, breed, etc.). PetFinder will then display a match of your choices, including photos and basic information about adoptable pets in shelters close to your home.

To learn more about how a rescued pet can make a positive difference in the lives of others, visit this guide's Web site, www. LivingAtTheEndOfLife.com.

❧ APPENDIX B ❧

Important Documents to Gather

Following is a list of documents you will find helpful to have available at this time. If the documents are located in a safe deposit box, move them to a more accessible but secure location, such as a lockbox within your home, or with a trusted loved one.

- Advance Directive and Medical Power of Attorney forms
- Birth certificate
- Social Security card
- Marriage certificate
- Divorce decree
- Military service discharge papers
- Naturalization/immigration papers
- Adoption papers
- Long-term care insurance policy
- Health insurance policy
- Life insurance policies
- Property, motor vehicle, and other insurance policies
- Will
- Checking, savings, and retirement account information
- Titles and deeds to property (including motor vehicles)
- Prearranged burial or cremation paperwork
- Federal, state, and other tax records for the past seven years
- Financial information, including loans, outstanding debts, business agreements, and other important financial documents
- Combinations or keys to a safe or lock box
- List and location of items stored or loaned
- User IDs or log-in names and passwords to online accounts
- Credit card information
- Names and contact information for your accountant, attorney, financial advisor, or other professionals

❧ Appendix C ❧

Common Pain Medications

Common Pain Medications	Is it timed-release?	How long will it last?	How soon will you feel the full effect?	Is there a need for laxatives?	
Short Acting					
Tylenol # 3 (300/30)*(1)	No	3–4 hours	1 hour	Yes	
Percocet (2.5/325)*(1)	No	3–4 hours	1 hour	Yes	
Percocet (5/325)*(1)	No	3–4 hours	1 hour	Yes	
Percocet (7.5/500)*(1)	No	3–4 hours	1 hour	Yes	
Percocet (10/650)*(1)	No	3–4 hours	1 hour	Yes	
Vicodin (5/500)*(1)	No	3–4 hours	1 hour	Yes	
Vicodin ES (7.5/750)*(1)	No	3–4 hours	1 hour	Yes	
Morphine/MSIR Tablets	No	3–4 hours	1 hour	Yes	
Morphine Liquid/Roxanol	No	3–4 hours	1 hour	Yes	
Oxycodone/Roxicodone	No	3–4 hours	1 hour	Yes	
Oxycodone Liquid/Oxyfast	No	3–4 hours	1 hour	Yes	
Hydromorphone/Dilaudid	No	3–4 hours	1 hour	Yes	
Long Acting					
MS-Contin/Oramorph SR	Yes	8–12 hours	Continuous *(3)	Yes	
Oxycontin	Yes	8–12 hours	Continuous *(3)	Yes	
Methadone	No	8 hours	1 hour	Yes	
Fentanyl/Duragesic Patch	Yes	48–72 hours	Continuous *(4)	Yes	

*Note *(1)   Effective January 2014, the US Food and Drug Administration will limit the amount of acetaminophen in Tylenol #3, Percocet, Vicodin, and other medication. If you are prescribed or are taking an over-the-counter medicine that contains acetaminophen (also known as Tylenol) ask your pharmacist or health care team how many tablets you can take in 24 hours.*

Can it be crushed and absorbed in the mouth?	Can it be given rectally?	Is there a limit of how many in 24 hours?	Is there a limit of how many in 24 hours if liver impaired?	Is there a limit of how many in 24 hours if kidney impaired?
Yes	Yes	Yes–13 tabs	8 tabs or fewer	Yes–13 tabs
Yes	Yes	Yes–12 tabs	7 tabs or fewer	Yes–12 tabs
Yes	Yes	Yes–12 tabs	7 tabs or fewer	Yes–12 tabs
Yes	Yes	Yes–8 tabs	5 tabs or fewer	Yes–8 tabs
Yes	Yes	Yes–6 tabs	3 tabs or fewer	Yes–6 tabs
Yes	Yes	Yes–8 tabs	5 tabs or fewer	Yes–8 tabs
Yes	Yes	Yes–5 tabs	3 tabs or fewer	Yes–5 tabs
Yes	Yes	No limit	No limit	Do not take *(2)
Yes–liquid	No	No limit	No limit	Do not take *(2)
Yes	Yes	No limit	No limit	No limit
Yes–liquid	No	No limit	No limit	No limit
Yes	Yes	No limit	No limit	No Limit
No	Yes	No limit	No limit	Do not take *(2)
No	Yes	No limit	No limit	No limit
Yes	Yes-tabs only	No limit	No limit	No limit
No	No	No *(5)	No *(5)	No *(5)

Note *(2)   *Morphine use with impaired kidney function can lead to toxicity.*

Note *(3)   *First dose onset approximately 6 hours, then subsequent doses continuous.*

Note *(4)   *First dose onset approximately 8–12 hours, then subsequent doses continuous.*

Note *(5)   *Maximum effective dose for the Fentanyl/Duragesic transdermal patches is 300 mcg.*

❈ Appendix D ❈

Supportive Therapies

In recent years an increasing number of families have sought additional therapies, such as acupuncture, guided imagery, massage, and supplements to complement their medical treatment. Instead of surgical or pharmacological (medication) interventions, many of these therapies utilize a variety of techniques to engage the individual's inner resources. These therapies offer great promise in that they may provide some degree of symptom relief and promote a sense of whole-body well-being, while having few or no side effects. Many treatments also offer benefit to families by providing a greater opportunity to participate with care and, as self-care, offer some relief from the physical, emotional, and spiritual symptoms that may result from the multiple stresses associated with caregiving and loss.

Though many of these therapies have been practiced for centuries, rigorous scientific research on their effectiveness did not begin until recently. Research in this field is especially challenging—in part because of lack of funding, but also because of the unique nature of these therapies, which often involve the mind as well as the body in the healing process. In many cases, conventional testing models simply do not apply, and researchers and practitioners have yet to reach consensus on effective methods to test and measure the effects of these nonconventional therapies.

But there is good news. Those of us who practice palliative and end-of-life care recognize the pressing need for useful information to support informed decision making among those we serve. For individuals and families facing a life-limiting illness, each day, each moment represents a choice: How do I spend the time I have left? What's the best use of the energy I have? If I spend my time and energy arranging for and receiving this treatment, will I feel better?

To help you make better-informed decisions, this appendix summarizes what is currently known about the effectiveness of the more widely available supportive therapies in relieving symptoms common at the end of life. The information is presented in two tables. The first table shows supportive therapies for specific symptoms. The second table shows supportive therapies for symptoms some caregivers may experience. Following these tables, you'll find a brief description of these therapies, and general precautions for each one.

Within each table you'll also find information about the state of the research for each therapy. In some cases, only limited pilot studies have been conducted. This level of evidence is described in this book as *investigational*. Another way to characterize this would be to say that we think this therapy *might* improve this symptom, but we're not sure. For those therapies that have benefited from several small- to midsized, well-designed studies, this level of evidence is described here as *fair*, meaning we feel there's a good chance that this therapy might improve the specified symptom, but, again, we're not sure. To be considered *conclusive*, large, well-designed clinical trials, using accepted methodology, must have been completed. For now, this appendix shares with you what is known, in hopes that this information is, in some way, useful to you. For emerging information, visit this book's Web site, www. LivingAtTheEndOfLife.com

To learn more about these therapies, talk with your hospice or health care provider. Many hospices and palliative care agencies can help you learn to perform these techniques at home, or help you locate a qualified practitioner. Before initiating any new therapies, consult your physician.

Be aware that herbs and supplements are a form of medication and can interact with your current medications or cause side effects. If you choose to consider herbs or supplements, consult your physician and discuss possible interactions and side effects.

Supportive Therapies for Symptoms Common at End of Life

Benefit	Therapy	Strength of Evidence	Footnote*
Short-Term Pain Relief	Massage	Fair	1, 2, 3, 4, 5, 6, 7
	Light Stroke Back Massage	Fair	1, 2, 8
	Foot Massage	Investigational	2, 9
	Light Touch Massage	Investigational	2
	Humor	Investigational	10
	Relaxation with Guided Imagery	Investigational	11, 12
	Music Therapy	Investigational	13
Decreased Nausea and/or Vomiting	Massage	Investigational	2, 4, 5
	Foot Massage	Investigational	2, 9
	Light Touch Massage	Investigational	2
	Relaxation with Guided Imagery	Investigational	11
Decreased Chemotherapy Induced Nausea and/or Vomiting	Acupuncture or Acupressure	Fair	14, 15
	Progressive Muscle Relaxation	Investigational	16, 17
	Relaxation with Guided Imagery	Investigational	18
	Ginger	Investigational	19
Decreased Fatigue	Massage	Investigational	2, 3, 5, 6
	Foot Massage	Investigational	2
	Light Touch Massage	Investigational	2
	Relaxation with Guided Imagery	Investigational	11
	Mindfulness Meditation	Investigational	20

*Information about footnotes is given in the bibliography on pages 227–231.

Benefit	Therapy	Strength of Evidence	Footnote
Decreased Fatigue with End-Stage Renal Disease	Acupressure	Investigational	21
Decreased Anxiety	Massage	Investigational	2, 4, 5, 7
	Foot Massage	Investigational	2
	Light Touch Massage	Investigational	2
	Reflexology	Investigational	22
	Relaxation with Guided Imagery	Investigational	11, 20
Decreased Depression	Massage	Investigational	2, 5, 23
	Foot Massage	Investigational	2
	Relaxation with Guided Imagery	Investigational	11
	Mindfulness Meditation	Investigational	20
Improved Sleep Quality	Massage	Investigational	6, 23
Increased Relaxation	Foot Massage	Investigational	9
	Relaxation with Guided Imagery	Investigational	11
	Mindfulness Meditation	Investigational	24
	Music Therapy	Investigational	13
Improved Mood	Relaxation with Guided Imagery	Investigational	11
	Mindfulness Meditation	Investigational	20, 24, 25
	Massage	Fair	1, 3
	Humor	Investigational	10

Supportive Therapies for Caregivers

Benefit	Therapy	Strength of Evidence	Footnote
Decreased Anxiety	Massage	Investigational	26
Improved Sleep	Massage	Investigational	27, 28
Decreased Depression	Massage	Investigational	26
Decreased Feelings of Stress	Massage	Investigational	27, 29
	Pet Companionship	Investigational	30, 31
Decreased Emotional and Physical Fatigue	Massage	Investigational	26, 27
Improved Mood	Massage	Investigational	29
Decreased Blood Pressure	Mindfulness Meditation	Investigational	32
	Pet Companionship	Investigational	33
	Humor	Investigational	10
Decreased Physical and Psychological Symptoms of Bereavement	Pet Companionship	Investigational	34
Decreased Depression Among Bereaved	Pet Companionship	Investigational	35
Improved Immune Function	Humor	Investigational	10
Increased Feelings of Helpfulness When Caring for a Loved One	Instruction in Massage	Investigational	36
Improved Health and Feeling of Well-Being	Healthy Diet	Conclusive	37

Description of Supportive Therapies Shown in the Tables

Acupuncture and Acupressure

The premise of acupuncture and acupressure is that energy flows in specific paths within our bodies, and acupuncture and acupressure, skillfully applied, can improve the flow of that energy. Acupuncture involves a specially trained, licensed practitioner inserting fine needles into specific points on the body to achieve a therapeutic effect. Similarly, acupressure involves a specially trained, licensed practitioner applying pressure to specific points on the body to achieve a therapeutic effect. In many cases, family members can be taught to correctly apply acupressure for specific purposes. *Cautions:* Acupuncture must be performed by a licensed professional. To locate a licensed practitioner in your community, talk with your hospice or health care team.

Ginger

The use of the ginger plant as a digestive aid dates back more than two thousand years. Commonly found in grocery stores as "gingerroot," it is also available in foods and beverages, such as cookies and tea. Ginger is also found in health food stores as a supplement in capsules or powders. *Cautions:* Ginger can interfere with the absorption or actions of medications, so talk with your physician before taking it. Ginger may interfere with blood clotting, so do not take it if you are on blood-thinning medications or have low blood platelets (less than 40,000). (Platelets are related to blood clotting. Low platelet levels may occur in people who have leukemia or HIV. Low platelet levels may also occur in people who have had chemotherapy or take blood-thinning medications.) Excessive use of ginger may cause heartburn, diarrhea, or irritation of the mouth. Ginger supplements are unregulated by the FDA and some products may contain contaminants. If you choose to take ginger, take only fresh ginger, foods or beverages prepared with real, not artificial ginger, or purchase supplements from a reliable manufacturer.

Guided Imagery

Guided imagery utilizes a person's own imagination to help her envision a different state of being. The premise of guided imagery is that the mind and body are connected, and the body will respond to what the mind believes is real. When used as a supportive therapy, the individual concentrates on pleasant images or memories, or an imagined, pleasant future state, and thus alters, to some extent, her body's response to its current situation. Guided imagery is often practiced with progressive muscle relaxation. In practicing these combined techniques, individuals focus first on relaxation. Once relaxation is achieved, they then utilize guided imagery to achieve a desired state of peace. *Cautions:* None

Healthy Diet and Appropriate Exercise for Caregivers

Though no studies have been conducted on the effects of a healthy diet and appropriate exercise on caregivers, studies on the general population have shown benefits in overall health and feelings of well-being. A healthy diet and appropriate exercise may be especially helpful during bereavement to reduce the physical symptoms of grief. Multiple studies have shown that a Mediterranean diet—a diet rich in vegetables, fruits, and whole grains, with minimal processed foods (sugar, white flour products, etc.)—offers significant health benefits. Studies show that exercise (appropriate to the individual's health and physical ability) improves health and may reduce a range of symptoms. Talk with your physician about what diet and exercise may be appropriate for you.

Humor

Humor needs no explanation. Laughter releases tension, fosters intimacy, and creates a series of positive physiological responses that we are only just beginning to understand. Perhaps most important, laughter enhances our ability to find meaning and courage in the face of seemingly insurmountable obstacles. *Cautions:* None

Massage

Massage therapy involves the application of touch to the body's soft tissues to achieve a therapeutic effect. Research has shown that massage, performed by an individual (such as a loved one, a friend, or a caregiver) who has been given some massage training, may be as effective at relieving symptoms as massage given by a licensed massage therapist. In general, only light or slow-stroke back massage, or foot massage, is appropriate for those who are not licensed massage therapists to perform. *Cautions:* Before beginning massage therapy, talk with your physician about any risks you might have.

Massage may *not* be appropriate if you have:

- Burns, rashes, or open wounds on the skin surface to be massaged.
- Unhealed broken bones in the limb or area to be massaged.
- Cancer invading your bones (bone metastasis).
- Cancerous tumors in the area to be massaged.
- Severe osteoporosis.
- Rheumatoid arthritis in the area (hand, foot, etc.) to be massaged.
- Blood clots (deep vein thrombosis).
- Experienced a recent heart attack.
- Low platelets (less than 40,000; see "Ginger Cautions" above).
- Swelling caused by cancer (lymphedema) in the limb to be massaged (it may be appropriate, however, if performed by a licensed massage therapist familiar with lymphedema; talk with your physician about your situation).

Meditation and Mindfulness-Based Stress Reduction

Meditation can be described as focusing the mind to promote a state of calmness, so the mind and body can be brought into greater harmony. Many techniques for meditation exist. The technique of mindfulness-based stress reduction involves experiencing thoughts, emotions, and sensations without judgment, with acceptance for the current state of being. *Cautions:* None.

Music Therapy

Music therapy involves the use of music to promote an improved state of being. It may involve either composed music or improvised tones to produce desired effects. Though commonly used in hospice care, to date, almost no research has been conducted on the effectiveness of music therapy. *Cautions:* None.

Pet Companionship

Pet companionship, as described in the studies, involves forming and maintaining a caring bond with a living, domestic animal, such as a dog, a cat, a rabbit, or another animal. *Cautions:* If you do not have a pet but are considering adopting one, evaluate your situation to make sure that you are able to provide care for the lifetime of the animal.

Progressive Muscle Relaxation

Progressive muscle relaxation utilizes focused breathing, combined with a technique of sequentially tensing then relaxing groups of muscles to achieve relaxation. The goal of this practice is to achieve an increased feeling of calm and a sense of inner peace. Progressive muscle relaxation is often practiced in conjunction with guided imagery. In practicing these combined techniques, individuals focus first on relaxation. Once relaxation is achieved, they then utilize guided imagery to achieve a desired state of peace. *Cautions:* None

Reflexology

Like acupuncture and acupressure, reflexology is based on the premise that energy flows in specific patterns within our body, and that energy can be manipulated for beneficial results. The practice of reflexology involves the application of massage to specific points on the body (often the feet, hands, or ears) to reduce symptoms and promote a sense of well-being. *But a word of caution:* Before beginning reflexology therapy, talk with your physician about any risks you might have. If your physician feels that reflexology is appropriate for you, arrange for a trained practitioner, familiar with your medical issues, to perform this therapy.

Reflexology may *not* be appropriate if you have:

- Burns, rashes, or open wounds on the skin surface to be touched.
- Unhealed broken bones in the extremity to be touched.
- Rheumatoid arthritis in the extremity to be touched.
- Blood clots (deep vein thrombosis).
- Infection in the extremity to be touched.
- Low platelets (less than 40,000; see "Ginger Cautions" above).

Bibliography for Table Footnotes

1. Kutner, J. S., Smith, M. C., Corbin, L., Hemphill, L., Benton, K., Mellis, K., Beaty, B., Felton, S, Yamashita, T. E., Bryant, L. L., Fairclough, D. L. "Massage therapy versus simple touch to improve pain and mood in patients with advanced cancer." *Annals of Internal Medicine,* 2008; 149(6): 369–379.
2. Cassileth, B. R., Vickers, A. J. "Massage therapy for symptom control: Outcome study at a major cancer center." *Journal of Pain and Symptom Management,* 2004; (28) 244–249.
3. Listing, M., Reibhauer, A., Krohn, M., Voigt, B., Tjahono, G., Becker, J., Klapp, B. F., Rauchfub, M. "Massage therapy reduces physical discomfort and improves mood disturbances in women with breast cancer." *Psycho-Oncology,* February 2009.
4. Wilkinson, S., Barnes, K., Storey, L. "Massage for symptom relief in patients with cancer: Systematic review." *Journal of Advanced Nursing,* 2008; 63(5): 430–439.
5. Ernst, E. "Massage therapy for cancer palliation and supportive care: a systematic review of randomized clinical trials." *Support Care in Cancer,* January 13, 2009; 17(4): 333-337.
6. Smith, M. C., Kemp, J., Hemphill, L., Vojir, C. P. "Outcomes of therapeutic massage for hospitalized cancer patients." *Journal of Nursing Scholarship,* 2002; 34: 257–262.

7. Sui-Wai, J., Wilkie, D., Gallucci, B., Beaton, R., Huang, H. "Effects of full body massage on pain intensity, anxiety, and psychological relaxation in Taiwanese patients with metastatic bone pain: A pilot study." *Journal of Pain and Symptom Management,* 2009; 37(4): 754–763.

8. Weinrich, S., Weinrich, M. "The effect of massage on pain in cancer patients." *Applied Nursing Research,* 1990; 3: 140–145.

9. Grealish, L., Lomasney, A., Whitman, B. "Foot massage: A nursing intervention to modify the distressing symptoms of pain and nausea in patients hospitalized with cancer." *Cancer Nursing,* 2000; 23: 237–243.

10. Christie, W., Moore, C. "The impact of humor on patients with cancer." *Clinical Journal of Oncology Nursing,* 2005, 9(2): 211–218.

11. Luebbert, K., Dahme, B., Hassenbring, M. "The effectiveness of relaxation training in reducing treatment related symptoms and improving emotional adjustment in acute non-surgical cancer treatment: A meta-analytical review." *Psycho-Oncology,* 2001; 10: 490–502.

12. Kwekkeboom, K., Wanta, B., Bumpas, M. "Individual difference variables and the effects of progressive muscle relaxation and analgesic imagery interventions on cancer pain." *Journal of Pain and Symptom Management,* 2008; 36(6): 604–615.

13. Krout, R. E. "The effects of single-session music therapy interventions on the observed and self-reported levels of pain control, physical discomfort and relaxation of hospice patients." *American Journal of Hospice and Palliative Care,* 2001; 18(6): 383–390.

14. Ezzo, J., Vickers, A., Richardson, M. A., Allen, C., Dibble, S. L., Issell, B., Lao, L., Pearl, M., Ramirez, G., Roscoe, J. A., Shen, J., Shivnan, J., Streitberger, K., Treish, I., Zangh, G. "Acupuncture-point stimulation for chemotherapy induced nausea and vomiting." Cochrane Database Systematic Review, April 19, 2006; (2) CD002285, and *Journal of Clinical Oncology,* 2005; 23(28): 7188–7198.

15. Lee, J., Dodd, M., Dibble, S., Abrams, D. "Review of acupressure studies for chemotherapy induced nausea and vomiting control." *Journal of Pain and Symptom Management,* 2008; 36(5): 529–522.

16. Arakawa, S. "Relaxation to reduce nausea, vomiting, and anxiety induced by chemotherapy in Japanese patients." *Cancer Nursing,* 1997; 20: 342–349.

17. Molassiotis, A. "A pilot study of the use of progressive muscle relaxation training in the management of post-chemotherapy nausea and vomiting." *European Journal of Cancer Care,* 2008; 9(4): 230–234.

18. Troesch, L. M., Rodehaver, C. B., Delaney, E. A., Yanes, B. "The influence of guided imagery on chemotherapy-related nausea and vomiting." *Oncology Nursing Forum,* 1993; 8: 1179–1185.

19. Ernst, E., Pittler, M. H. "Efficacy of ginger for nausea and vomiting: A systematic review of randomized controlled trials." *British Journal of Anaesthesia,* 2000; 84(3): 367–371.

20. Speca, M., Carlson, L., Goodey, E., Angen, M. "A randomized wait-list controlled clinical trial: The effect of a mindfulness meditation-based stress reduction program on mood and symptoms of stressing cancer outpatients." *Psychosomatic Medicine,* 2000; 62: 613–622.

21. Tsay, S. L. "Acupressure and fatigue in patients with end-stage renal disease: A randomized controlled trial." *International Journal of Nursing Studies,* 2004; 41(1): 99–106.

22. Stephenson, N., Weinrich, S., Tavakoli, A. "The effects of foot reflexology on anxiety and pain in patients with breast and lung cancer." *Oncology Nursing Forum,* 2000; 27: 67–72.

23. Soden, K., Vincent, K., Craske, S., Lucas, C., Ashley, S. "A randomized controlled trial of aromatherapy massage in a hospice setting." *Palliative Medicine,* 2004; 18(2): 87–92.

24. Smith, J. E., Richardson, J., Hoffman, C., Pilkington, K. "Mindfulness-Based Stress Reduction as supportive therapy in cancer care: A systematic review." *Journal of Advanced Nursing,* 2005; 52(3): 315–327.

25. Carlson, L. E., Ursuliak, Z., Goodey, E., Angen, M., Speca, M. "The effects of a mindfulness medication-based stress reduction program on mood and symptoms of stress in cancer outpatients: A 6-month follow-up." *Support Care Cancer,* 2001; 9(2): 112-123.

26. Rexilius, S., Mundt, C., Megel, M., Agrawal, S. "Therapeutic effects of massage therapy and healing touch on caregivers of patients undergoing autologous hematopoietic stem cell transplant." *Oncology Nursing Forum,* 2002; 29: E35-E44.

27. MacDonald, G. "Massage as a respite intervention for primary caregivers." *American Journal of Hospice and Palliative Care,* 1998; 15(1): 43-47.

28. Mackereth, P., Sylt, P., Weinberg, A., Campbell, G. "Chair massage for carers in an acute cancer hospital." *European Journal of Oncology Nursing,* 2005; 9(2): 167-179.

29. Goodfellow, L. M. "The effects of therapeutic back massage on psychophysiologic variables and immune function on spouses of patients with cancer." *Nursing Research,* 2003; 52(5): 318-328.

30. Allen, K., Blascovich, J., Mendes, W. B. "Cardiovascular reactivity and the presence of pets, friends and spouses: The truth about cats and dogs." *Psychosomatic Medicine,* 2002; 64(5): 727-739.

31. Allen, K., Blascovich, J., Tomaka, J., Kelsey, R. "Presence of human friends and pet dogs as moderators of autonomic responses to stress in women." *Journal of Personality and Social Psychology,* 1991; 61(4): 582-589.

32. Walton, K., Schneider, R., Nidich, S. "Review of controlled research on the transcendental meditation program and cardiovascular disease: Risk factors, morbidity and mortality." *Cardiology Review,* 2004; 12(5): 262-266.

33. Allen, K. "Dog ownership and control of borderline hypertension: A controlled randomized trial." Presented at the 22nd Annual Scientific Session of the Society of Behavioral Medicine, March 24, 2001, Seattle.

34. Akiyama, H., Holtzman, J. M., Britz, W. E. "Pet ownership and health

status during bereavement." *Omega Journal of Death and Dying,* 1987; 17(1): 87–93.

35. Garrity, T. F., Stallones, L., Marx, M. B., Johnson, T. P. "Pet ownership and attachment as supportive factors in the health of the elderly." *Anthrozoos,* 1989; 3(1): 35–44.

36. Collinge, W., Kahn, J., Yarold, P., Bauer-Wu, S., McCorkle, R. "Couples and cancer: Feasibility of brief instruction in massage and touch therapy to build caregiver efficacy." *Journal of the Society for Integrative Oncology,* 2007; 5(4): 147–154.

37. deLorgeril, M., Salen, P. "The Mediterranean diet: Rationale and evidence for its benefit," *Current Atherosclerosis Reports,* December 2008; 10(6): 518–522.

❧ ACKNOWLEDGMENTS ❧

We don't accomplish anything in this world alone . . . and whatever
happens is the result of the whole tapestry of one's life and all the weavings
of individual threads from one to another that creates something.

—Sandra Day O'Connor

Like a tapestry, this guide evolved through the contributions of many people. Their ideas, efforts, encouragement, and gentle wisdom were woven together, thread by thread, to create this guide.

Some of the threads are quite old, contributed by generations of nurses who came before me, who tenaciously pushed the social and institutional boundaries that previously defined nursing to create a profession that, today, offers far more than just compassionate presence.

Some of the threads are quite new, contributed by researchers in biomedicine, nursing, and social science. Their work continues to uncover better ways to address problems and improve quality of life.

Some of the threads simply blend in, yet they serve as a foundation, for they are woven in by teachers—in classrooms and in the workplace. These teachers recognize that the strength of one is nothing compared to the strength of many, and so they give, content to know that what they give will grow into something far greater, becoming part of the wider body of collective knowledge.

And, finally, this tapestry's true character comes from a multitude of threads, each with its own color and texture and meaning. These are the threads contributed by those whom I have met along the way, the individuals who faced their own death or that of someone they love. From you I have learned the most—about life, about living, about growth, hope, and healing.

Woven into this guide are also the contributions of many who gave their time, energy, and ideas to create this guide.

For Helping to Shape this Guide's Content (alphabetically):

Nancy Boutin, MD—for review of select chapters and valuable suggestions that significantly improved the format and readability

Louise Carroll—for review of the entire manuscript and helpful suggestions as you care for your parents

Loretta Clark, LCSW—for review of select chapters and helpful suggestions, and for being a standard bearer for hospice social work

Patrick Clary, MD—for permission to use your evocative poem, *Grief Work*

Jilly Eddy & Marsha Kremen—for reviewing the entire manuscript and offering helpful suggestions drawn from your experiences having cared for loved ones through this process, and for enlisting review by others facing this challenge

Barb Farmer, RN, CHPCA—for creating the flexibility for me to remain at H.H. while I developed this guide

Sue Farthing, CNA—for review of select chapters and helpful suggestions, and for your partnership during our years together at H.H.

Daniel Fischberg, MD, PhD—for helpful suggestions as I researched elements of this guide

Laird Goodman, DVM—for years of compassionate care—and end-of-life care—of another form

Milo Haas, RPh—for review of select chapters and helpful suggestions, and for serving as a mentor to me and so many others

Larry Hansen, MA, CT—for offering a chaplain's perspective and suggestions for select chapters, and for sharing the vision of what end-of-life care can be

Joan Harrold, MD, FAAHPM, MPH, and Joanne Lynn, MD—for permission to use material from your helpful book, *Handbook for Mortals*

Miles Hassell, MD—for helping to shape the Supportive Therapies appendix

Scott Irwin, MD, PhD—for unraveling prevention and treatment of delirium for me so that I could share useful information with families

Ed Israel—for your encouragement for this project, for review of select chapters and helpful suggestions, and for being a truly great friend!

Karen Kehl, RN, PhD, ACHPN—for your scholarship in end-of-life educational materials, and for review of Parts IV and V and helpful suggestions

Merritt Linn, MD—for your review of the entire manuscript and insightful editing, and for suggesting the title

Hob Osterlund, RN, MS—for information about the healing power of humor

Bobbie Paris & Jack Thornton—for review of the manuscript, and for placing it in Bonnie's hands

Beth Kei Ruml, RN, LCSW—for review of the entire manuscript, offering valuable suggestions as a long-time hospice nurse *and* social worker

Bonnie Saucier, PhD, RN—for review of the entire manuscript and helpful suggestions

Jan Seliken, RN, ND—for help researching the Supportive Therapies appendix

Rick Severson, PhD—for review of select chapters and helpful suggestions, and your calming presence for more than sixteen years as a Wednesday night volunteer at H.H.

Robert & Geraldine Swigart—for review of the entire manuscript and helpful suggestions as you face your own health challenges

Rick Warren, APRN, BC—for review of select chapters and helpful suggestions, and for begin a true leader

Ken Weizer, ND—for help in developing the Supportive Therapies appendix

The 2008 Board of the American Academy of Hospice & Palliative Medicine for awarding me a College of Palliative Care scholarship to support the development of this guide

Everyone at H.H. for being teachers and friends, special thanks to the Wednesday Night "Dream Team" Karen S., Sue, Deb, Rick, Barbara, and Tom, for all that you shared and taught me about teamwork and caring

For Helping to Transform This Idea into a Book (alphabetically)
Marilyn Allen of the Allen O'Shea Literary Agency—for sharing a vision
of compassion, and for efforts far beyond the line of duty; without your
belief in this message, this book would not have been possible
Michael Fragnito—for serving as a supportive executive sponsor
Elizabeth Mihaltse—for creating the evocative cover art
Dave Nelson—for believing in this message and building support so it
could reach families in need; best wishes on your journey
Kate Zimmermann—for serving as editor and navigator, striving to
bolster others in mind, body, and spirit
Everyone on the edit team, for your insights, suggestions, and thought
provoking questions; you greatly enriched this guide
Everyone at Sterling Publishing/Barnes & Noble—for the vision to
improve quality of life by sharing information through ease of access and
fair pricing practices

For Writing the Foreword
Dr. Charlie Sasser, MD, FAAHPM, FACP—Thank you for sharing your
insights, wisdom, grace, humility, and humor with me, and with those
who read this guide. I'm inspired by you, and am blessed to know you.

And My Family
My parents, Bob and Mary Whitley—for teaching me, through example,
to work hard for what I believe in.
And, most of all, thank you to Steve and our "kids" Holly, Biscuit, and
Zach—for reading, offering suggestions, and helping to craft this content
(or, in the case of the dogs, for napping beside me while I worked); and for
believing in me, for sharing every day, and for bringing joy to my life!
Thank you all. Without you this book would not have been possible.

Ackowledgments from Dr. Sasser
To Everyone at Sterling

Index

❄ ABOUT THE AUTHOR ❄

Karen Whitley Bell, RN, CHPN, has practiced as a hospice nurse since 1994, helping families find comfort and quality of life. She participates nationally in efforts to promote access and improve end-of-life care. She volunteers internationally, teaching end-of-life care and supporting microfinance initiatives to alleviate poverty. She lives in the Pacific Northwest, and is happiest when enjoying the company of friends and sharing long walks with her family on wooded mountain trails and along the rugged Pacific coast.

Charles G. Sasser, MD, FAAHPM, FACP, has been practicing medicine in his hometown of Conway, South Carolina for 35 years. He is a founding member and past president of the American Academy of Hospice and Palliative Medicine. When he is not reflecting on the amazing observations of his six grandchildren, he divides his professional time between the private practice of Internal Medicine, hospital-based Palliative Medicine, and community-based Mercy Hospice.